NEW DEVELOPMENTS IN MEDICAL RESEARCH

PICTORIAL ESSAYS ON PERITONEAL METASTASES IMAGING

CT, MRI AND PET-CT

NEW DEVELOPMENTS IN MEDICAL RESEARCH

Additional books and e-books in this series can be found on Nova's website under the Series tab.

NEW DEVELOPMENTS IN MEDICAL RESEARCH

PICTORIAL ESSAYS ON PERITONEAL METASTASES IMAGING

CT, MRI AND PET-CT

PAUL H. SUGARBAKER
AND
RUSSELL N. LOW
EDITORS

nova
Medicine & Health
New York

Library of Congress Cataloging-in-Publication Data

Names: Sugarbaker, Paul H., editor. Title: Pictorial essays on peritoneal metastases imaging : CT, MRI and PET-CT / Paul H. Sugarbaker, editor. Description: New York : Nova Science Publishers, [2020] | Series: New developments in medical research | Includes bibliographical references and index. | Summary: "Peritoneal metastases continue to be a potentially lethal manifestation of gastrointestinal and gynecologic malignancy. In the past little if any treatments except systemic chemotherapy were available. Outcomes of treatment were poor and were routinely regarded as palliative. This dismal outlook has gradually changed as a result of two technical innovations: 1) Cytoreductive surgery with peritonectomy procedures and visceral resections and 2) Perioperative intraperitoneal and systemic chemotherapy. At this time approximately 2000 peritoneal oncology centers are active around the globe. With prevention and treatment of peritoneal metastases a reality the traditional role of the radiologist to characterize the malignancy is mandatory for knowledgeable management. We have discovered that the radiologic description of peritoneal metastases is challenging, to say the least. Progress has occurred. In our Pictorial Essays on Peritoneal Metastases Imaging: CT, MRI and PET-CT our radiologists have gathered together an abundance of information. Our book has established a role of the radiologist as an essential part of multidisciplinary management of a common and complex clinical problem. No longer is the radiologist's role only to determine if peritoneal metastases are absent versus present. The best technology or combinations of technology as CT, MRI or PET-CT must be selected. Not only a diagnosis of peritoneal metastases but extent and distribution of disease is required. The oncologist and surgeon need to know the likelihood of success with treatment. For primary cancer identification of patients at high risk for local-regional recurrence allows special treatments to be utilized before treatment failure occurs. If recurrent disease is suspect, the radiologist may interpret its causation and describe the interventions required to treat or suggest only palliation. The associated features of peritoneal metastases such as ascites or lymphadenopathy must be interpreted. The report must be complete with all information required by the clinician. Finally, the knowledgeable quantitation of concerning radiologic features can have profound prognostic implications. Our book not only verbally describes the images of peritoneal metastases, it shows them in carefully selected radiographs. The figures, figure legends and text allow the findings to be interpreted so they are clinically relevant. The images become a visible guide to construct a management plan. The radiologist's accurate description of peritoneal metastases is difficult at best, sometimes impossible, but comprehensively presented in this book. If one is interested in peritoneal metastases, the Pictorial Essays on Peritoneal Metastases Imaging: CT, MRI and PET-CT is a required addition to the personal library"-- Provided by publisher. Identifiers: LCCN 2020020534 (print) | LCCN 2020020535 (ebook) |
ISBN 9781536180145 (paperback) | ISBN 9781536180152 (adobe pdf) Subjects: LCSH: Peritoneum--Cancer--Imaging.
Classification: LCC RC280.P38 P53 2020 (print) | LCC RC280.P38 (ebook) | DDC 616.99/465--dc23
LC record available at https://lccn.loc.gov/2020020534
LC ebook record available at https://lccn.loc.gov/2020020535

Published by Nova Science Publishers, Inc. † New York

CONTENTS

PREFACE

On 17-19 November 2016, the 10th International Congress on Peritoneal Surface Malignancies was held in Washington, DC. As a post-conference satellite symposium, a series of presentations regarding peritoneal metastases imaging occurred. Radiologists at prominent centers for the management of peritoneal metastases presented their extensive experience. This included Clarisse Dromain who was, at that time, lead radiologist for the Gustave Roussy Cancer Institute in Villejuif, France. James S. Jelinek is the chief of radiology at MedStar Washington Hospital Center in Washington, DC. Gina Brown is stationed at the Royal Marsden Cancer Institute in London and has been active in the peritoneal metastases work throughout the United Kingdom. Pascal Rousset is the lead peritoneal metastases radiologist at Lyon-Sud University Hospital in Lyon, France.

These presentations are the core material in our attempt to bring together the radiology of peritoneal metastases. This immense amount of clinical material was then extensively edited by myself and Russell Low and then returned to our radiologic world's experts for their editions, deletions, and further clarifications. These pictorial essays have undergone a 3-year process of being continually updated and revised. The radiologic technology has not changed over these many months but the importance of CT, MRI and PET-CT in the management of peritoneal metastases has continued to increase. Unless major innovations in radiologic technology occur, this textbook describes state-of-the-art imaging for peritoneal metastases for the next decade.

The book starts off with Clarisse Dromain's chapter calling for a standardization of the best technology of CT, MRI and PET-CT for peritoneal metastases. Her requirements for an optimal study are comprehensive but necessary in order to develop a complete report. Then, James Jelinek introduces the concept of the concerning radiologic features that are essential to the interpretation of the images acquired in peritoneal metastases patients. Concerning radiologic features may have a profound impact on patient management, and he suggests that quantitation of these concerning features is possible. Gina Brown takes a full step towards improving the management of primary colorectal cancer through the application of best radiologic principles for clinical judgments in the management of primary disease. It follows directly that these radiologic principles will assist in the early detection of recurrent disease. Pascal Rousset describes what can be learned from a study of peritoneal metastases by MRI. Then, Gina Brown uses CT, MRI and PET-CT to interpret surgical treatment failures in rectal cancer and radiologically describes the mechanism for recurrent disease. Clarisse Dromain establishes that peritoneal metastases are not an oncologic entity into themselves but have important associated clinical features. Then, Pascal Rousset lays out the report that is required for an adequate description of the patient's condition. Finally, James Jelinek jumps ahead of all previous work with the radiology of malignant peritoneal mesothelioma and establishes that the CT has profound prognostic information for the multidisciplinary team to evaluate preoperatively.

This book contains an abundance of information regarding the imaging of peritoneal metastases. Much of this information is not published elsewhere! We think this book is essential to all radiologists and oncologists who participate in the management of peritoneal metastases. This comprehensive radiologic description of peritoneal metastases may in the future evolve into a peritoneal metastases reporting and data system (PM-RADS). Our book is the first step in the formulation of such an important and badly needed systemized approach. As a surgeon and radiologist dedicated to the optimal management of peritoneal metastases, we believe it is imperative that the wealth of knowledge collected by our radiologists be preserved. Imaging of peritoneal metastases by CT, MRI and PET-CT and its application in the treatment of peritoneal metastases is challenging, but as these works clearly demonstrate, progress is being made.

Paul H. Sugarbaker, MD
Russell N. Low, MD

ACKNOWLEDGMENTS

The authors wish to thank Dr. Renaldo Savady for his tireless and indispensable work in the successful completion of this project. He succeeded in the original correlation of the text with 119 figures and 10 tables. He maintained the work electronically through three years of multiple revisions. Through his efforts a successful publication by Nova Science Publishers is now possible.

In: Pictorial Essays … ISBN: 978-1-53618-014-5
Editors: PH Sugarbaker and RN Low ©2020 Nova Science Publishers, Inc.

Chapter 1

Standardization of Best Technology of CT, MRI, and PET for Peritoneal Metastases

Clarisse Dromain, MD, PhD
University Hospital CHUV, Lausanne, Switzerland

Introduction

Imaging of peritoneal metastases is always a challenge. It is probably most difficult when we deal with gastrointestinal malignancy. First, this is a technical challenge because we must have imaging with a very high spatial resolution. This is because tumor nodules or plaques on peritoneal surfaces may be of very small size. Second, we must have a high contrast resolution because most tumor implants have a similar attenuation to small bowel wall and normal tissue. Also, often peritoneal implants have no significant enhancement with intravenous CT contrast. Third, we need a technology that minimizes motion artifact, in particular movement of the diaphragm and the small bowel. This is more important for PET-CT and MRI than CT, because the new generation of CT scanners are able to complete the abdominal and pelvic examination in a few seconds. Fourth, accurate interpretation is a challenge. We know that a major problem with the radiology of peritoneal metastases is inter-reader variability. If you compare sensitivity between readers, it can be very different from one to another. Sometimes we have a low confidence because of a high frequency of doubtful lesions. Too often peritoneal metastases are identified only in retrospect. This is not of helpful for treatment planning!

So what is the radiologist asked to provide? Not only are we asked to make a diagnosis of peritoneal dissemination but we also need to determine the extent and distribution of the disease. We know that the extent and distribution within the abdomen and pelvis of the peritoneal metastases is crucial for patient selection for treatment. This occurs because partial surgical removal of large volume tumor at a crucial anatomic site is associated with a high morbidity and is only of palliative benefit. Long term favorable results only accompany complete resection of all visible disease. Distribution is a prognostic factor. We must identify tumor present at crucial anatomic sites that are high-risk locations for complete cytoreduction [1]. This may be one of our most crucial tasks as a radiologist. For example, critical anatomic sites are tumor that involves the small bowel and its mesentery, structures of the porta hepatis, stomach and left gastric vessels, and extensive pelvic sidewall invasion. We need to mention the presence of tumor at these specific locations in our report. Finally, we must alert the clinician to extraperitoneal disease, if present.

CT as a Reference Imaging Modality

Every multidisciplinary team (MDT) requires a CT before surgery for peritoneal metastases for all patients. It is a useful examination, but it does have limitations. The per patient sensitivity regarding peritoneal metastases present versus absent was acceptable at 82%. In contrast, lesion by lesion sensitivity was quite low. In our study of 30 patients performed in 2008, the extent of the peritoneal dissemination was overestimated in 1 patient using CT. The extent of the peritoneal dissemination was underestimated in 21 patients (70%) using CT [2]. Finally, when we compared CT with PET-CT, the results were similar.

The sensitivity of CT examination depends not only on lesion size but also on the location of the peritoneal implant. It is quite good for epigastrium, left subphrenic space and periumbilical area, but lower accuracy in the pelvis, visceral peritoneum, and right subphrenic space. As might be expected, the size of tumor cell implant has a large influence on the sensitivity of CT. Implants more than 1 cm in size are usually well detected (Table 1.1.) [3-8].

Finally, radiologic expertise is a crucial point. In the study by Warde, 3 different radiologists produced a sensitivity ranging from 30-73% [9]. In the study by Coakley, Cohen's Kappa statistic was used to estimate the agreement among radiologists. The agreement with the Kappa ranged from 0.35 to 0.50 for peritoneal thickening assessment and very low 0.12-0.25 for small bowel involvement [10]. These data indicate that there is a real problem with interpretation between radiologists and a high inter-reader variability.

One of the major limitations of the CT assessment of peritoneal metastases is detection errors. This means that the implant or lesion was present in the CT images but the radiologist did not recognize it and did not report it. This is surprising since we now use multi-detector CT which is very fast with thin slices. Unfortunately, there is no significant increase in the sensitivity of peritoneal metastases detection with the use of advanced technology that allows 3D multiplanar reconstruction. Why? Because spatial resolution may not be the problem. In Figure 1.1 top and middle shows nodules that were present but not detected. The problem is contrast resolution. Most tumor implants have the same contrast as the normal adjacent tissue. One lesson we learned from PET-CT is that bright tracer uptake of peritoneal metastases may allow us to find tumor nodules retrospectively on CT after we initially missed them. The radiologist must remember that in some patients, especially thin patients, and those with no ascites, locations such as the mesentery, small bowel, and pelvis are frequent causes of detection errors. Figure 1 at the bottom shows a lesion in the pelvis that was not detected.

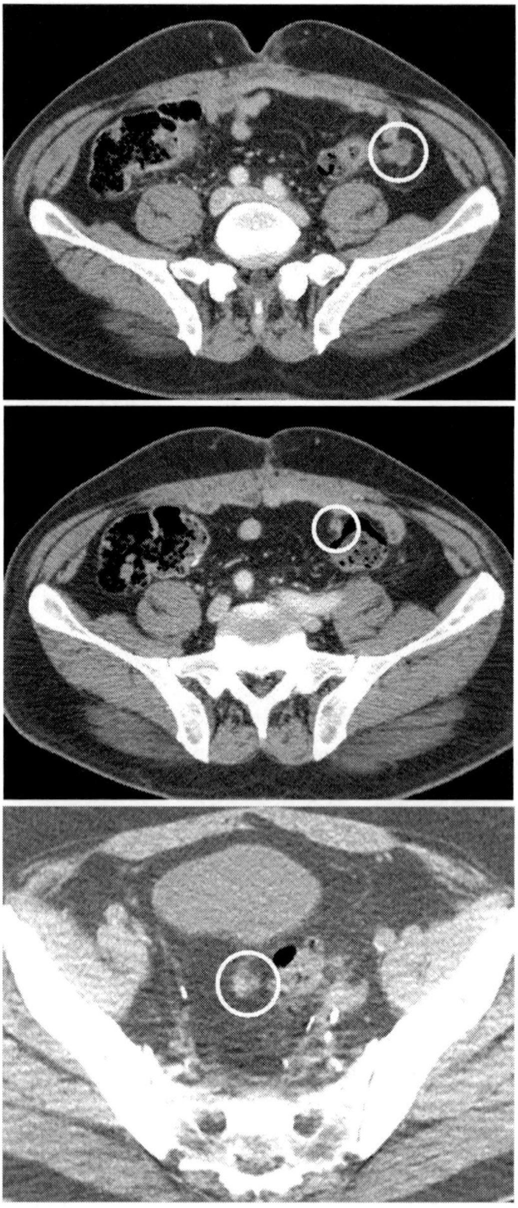

Figure 1.1. (top, middle and bottom). Missed peritoneal implants on axial CT images later confirmed to be cancerous. Although the implants are large in size they were missed due to the low contrast resolution of CT imaging and their similar appearance to adjacent small bowel.

Table 1.1. Sensitivity of CT to detect peritoneal metastases

Author	Year	Institution	No. of Patients	Detection > 1 cm	Detection < 0.5 cm
Jacquet	1993	Washington Cancer Institute, Washington, DC	45	79%	28%
Davies	1997	General Infirmary, Leeds, UK	17	71%	NA
De Bree	2004	Antoni van Leeuwenhoek, Amsterdam	25	60-76%	9-24%
Koh	2009	St. George Hospital, Sydney	19	60%	11%
Kim	2009	Seoul National University	53	28.3%	15
Marin	2010	University of Rome, Sapienza	18	75%	43%

NA = not available.

Another limitation of CT is interpretation errors. A good example of this is distinguishing a parenchymal liver metastases from a subdiaphragmatic implant. When a multiplanar reconstruction is performed, one sees that it is not a liver metastases but in actuality a peritoneal implant deeply indenting the liver parenchyma. There is also misinterpretation of peritoneal metastases versus lymph nodes, particularly within the small bowel mesentery. This is a common cause of error in both CT and PET-CT. Also, it may be difficult to distinguish between peritoneal metastases and spleen metastases. The hilum of the spleen is an area at special risk for the progression of peritoneal implants. Even though the spleen is grossly involved the lesion should not be misinterpreted as hematogenous metastases. Particularly, colorectal cancer peritoneal metastases involving the hilum of the spleen are more frequent than are hematogenous or lymphatic metastases. Also, an accessory spleen may be confused with a nodular left upper quadrant peritoneal metastasis.

To minimize the detection and interpretation errors by CT, we need high x- and z-spatial resolution. This enables the detection of smaller size implants. Axial spatial resolution needs to have adapted field of view and a high matrix.

Longitudinal spatial resolution requires small slice thickness. It is no longer a problem with our current CT scan machines. We also need fast breath-hold slice acquisition to minimize the motion artifacts caused by the diaphragm motion and peristalsis. We need to have minimal noise in images to increase the contrast to noise ratio.

With current scan technology we have the possibility to use different reconstruction algorithms. I think it is very useful to use a very low noise iterative reconstruction algorithm, in particular, for the fat. If you want to be able to see small deposits in the fat, we must have very low noise in our CT images. Finally, we need to have slice thickness reconstruction. I see this as a use for 3D reconstruction. As we search for peritoneal metastases in coronal and sagittal planes, we increase our possibility of detection.

If we want to be able to have a good quality 3D reconstruction we need to have thin slices. But for the interpretation of the axial plane, we need to have thicker slices to be able to increase the contrast. Figure 1.2 shows the same patient with different slice thickness reconstructions, 1 mm and 5 mm. You can see the quality of the 1 mm thickness is superior as compared to 5 mm where everything is blurred. If we don't perform thin slices, we will not be able to have a high quality of reconstruction. However, for interpretation it is better to have greater slice thickness which produce images with higher contrast and less noise. If you look at the fat you will be able to detect tumor implants more readily. So we need both – the thin slices to make the reconstruction and thick slices for the interpretation of images.

In Figure 1.3, there are two different scans in the same patient. The diagnosis is a recurrent pseudomyxoma and these CT scans were performed within a six-month interval with this slow growing tumor. You can see that we use two different generations of CT and two different algorithms for reconstruction. Once again, the noise in the fat is not the same and if you lower the standard deviation of attenuation using good iterative algorithm, it results in less noisy and better CT images.

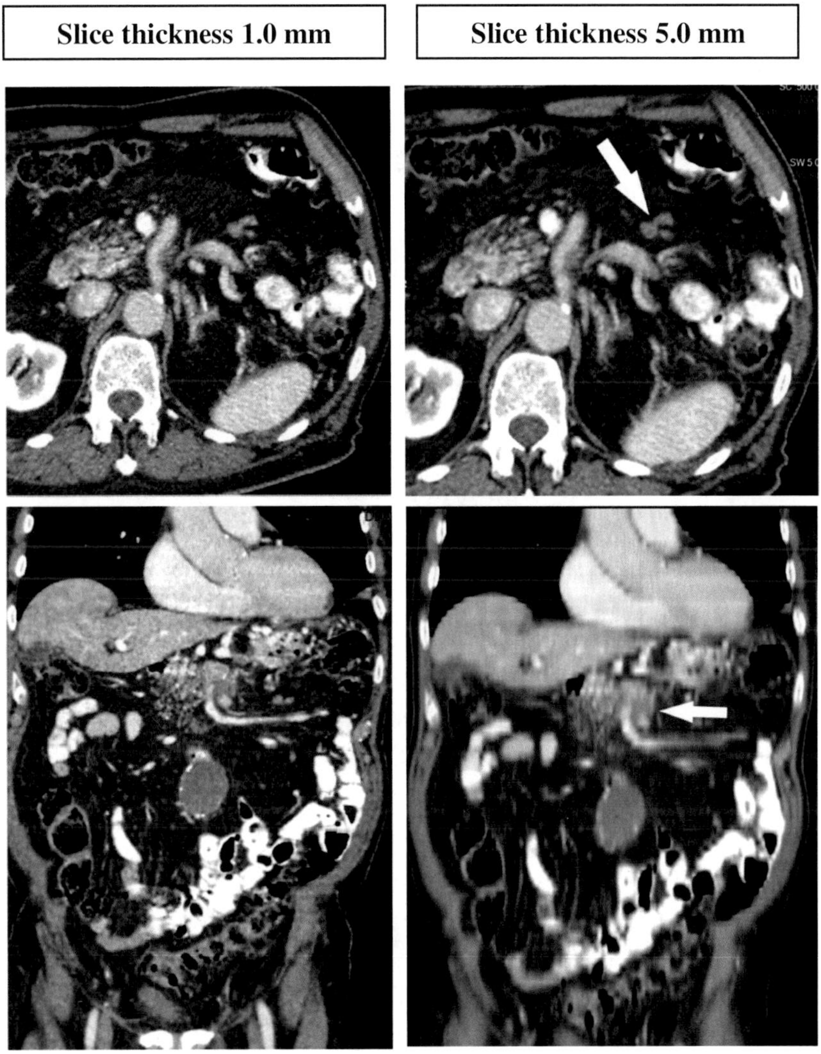

Figure 1.2. Difference of image quality depending upon acquisition parameter. Thin slice thickness of 1 mm is required to have a high quality in 3D reconstruction illustrated in this example in the coronal plane. However, the image noise is higher in thin slice than in thick leading to a decreased signal to noise ratio and so decreased detectability. To recover higher signal to noise ratio it is recommended to thicken the slice thickness from 1 mm to 2.5 to 5.0 mm for interpretation.

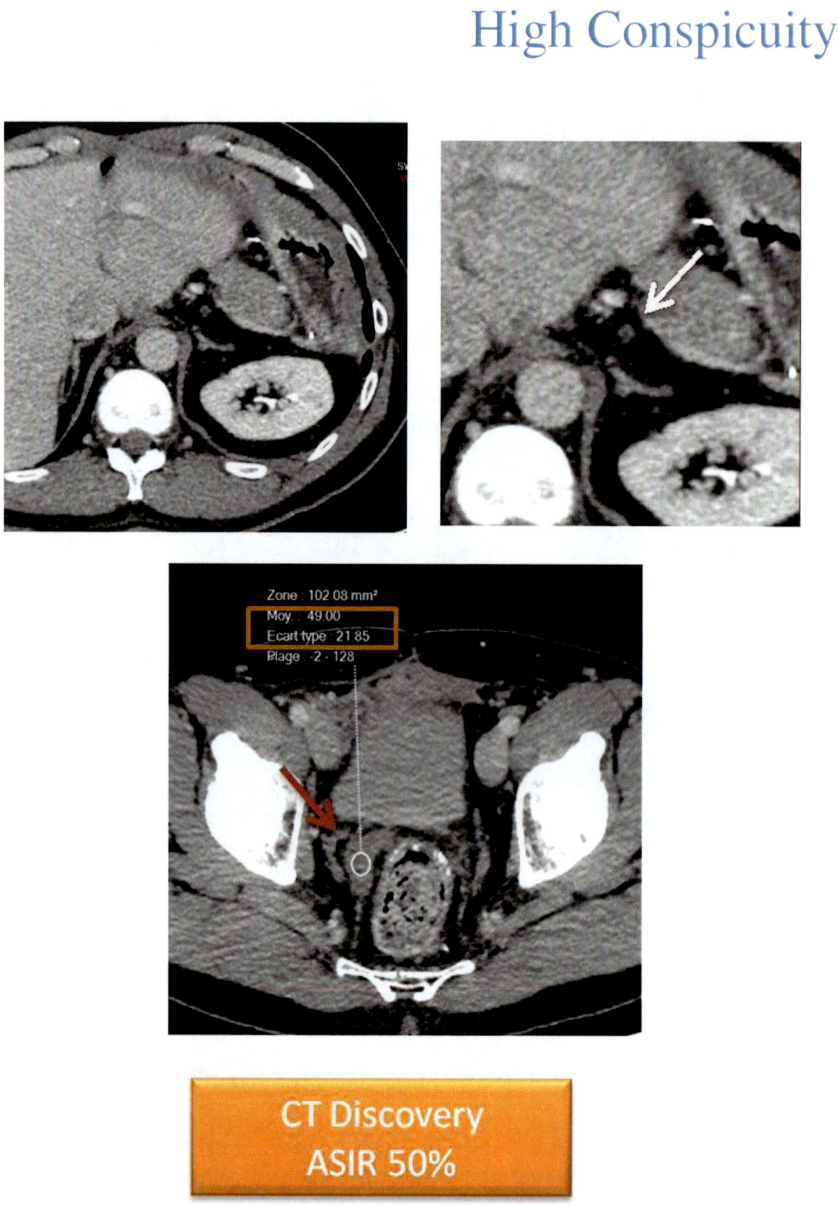

Figure 1.3. Influence of algorithm used in CT image reconstruction on image quality. CT images of the same patient using 2 different reconstruction algorithms. (Left side) Images acquired in a CT scan Discovery (GE Healthcare) reconstructed with ASIR 50% show higher noise (density SD: 21.85).

Due to low noise

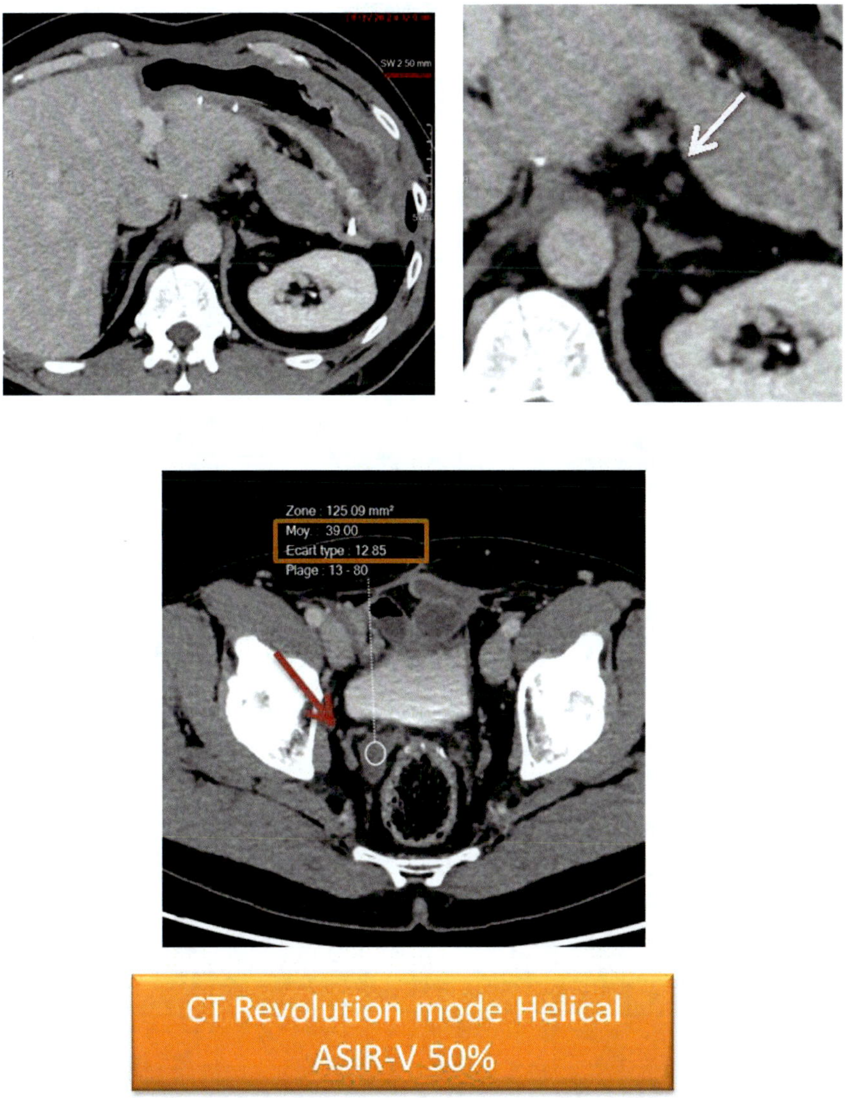

Figure 1.3 (Right side) Images acquired in a CT scan Revolution (GE Healthcare) reconstructed with ASIR-V 50% (density SD: 12.85).

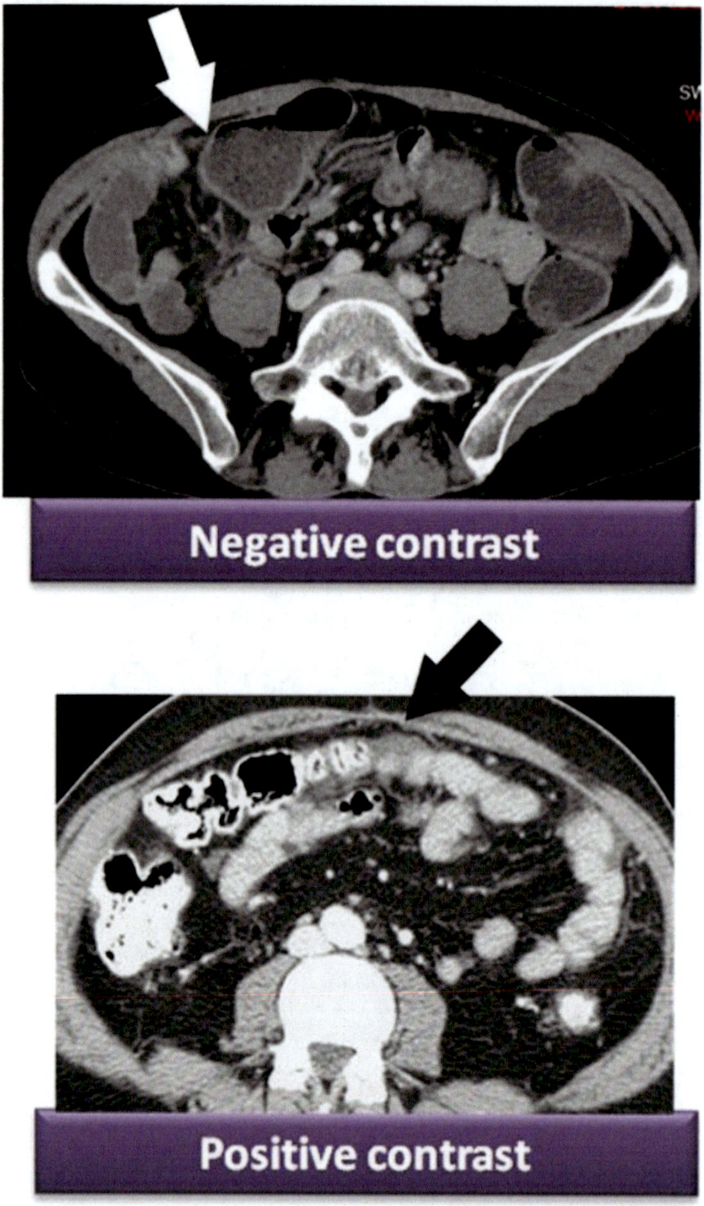

Figure 1.4. (top and bottom). Axial CT images with opacification of the small bowel by two different oral contrast. Involvement of the visceral peritoneum shown at the top (arrows) is not as well depicted using negative contrast (black) than using positive contrast shown at the bottom (white) due to the higher contrast to noise ratio between tumoral deposit and the small bowel wall.

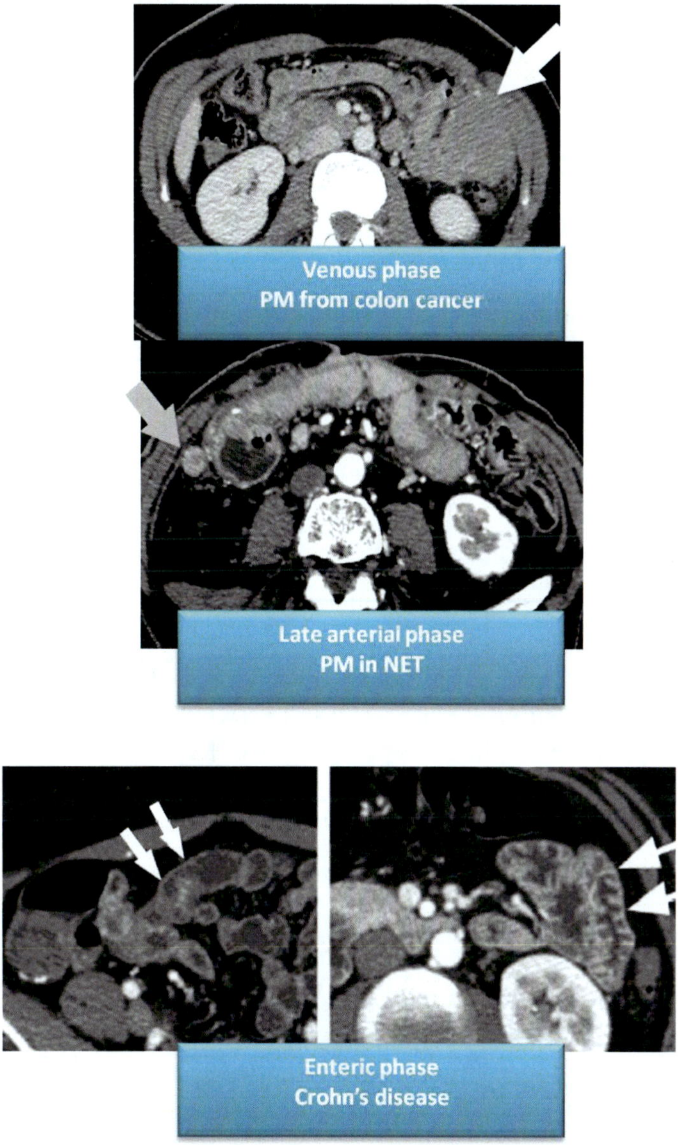

Figure 1.5. (top, middle and bottom). Axial CT images acquired at different times after the injection of intravenous contrast agent. The venous phase (70-90 seconds) is the regular phase for the detection of peritoneal metastases (top). The arterial phase (30 seconds) is mandatory only in cases of PM from hypervascularized tumors such as neuroendocrine tumor (middle). The enteric phase (45 seconds) has been shown to display the higher contrast of the small bowel wall enhancement in Crohn disease (bottom). However, its value for PM detection is unknown.

An effective CT methodology to reduce errors of detection and interpretation is the use of oral contrast. This increases our ability to visualize sub-centimetric deposits on small bowel serosa. We can use either positive or negative contrast. Tap water is the most commonly used negative contrast agent. Just half an hour before the CT, the patient has to rapidly drink about 1 liter of water. It provides improved delineation of the contrast-enhanced small bowel mucosa in comparison with the hypodense lumen. As shown in Figure 1.4 (top), the wall of the small bowel is depicted in contrast to the intraluminal water and does not produce beam-hardening artifact. In Figure 1.4 (bottom), positive contrast distinguishes between serosal deposits that are hypodense and the lumen of the small bowel defined by Barium or Iodine. One must remember that positive contrast limits identification of calcified peritoneal deposits and can obscure mucosal enhancement and the assessment of some subtle mural disease.

Again, in an effort to reduce errors of detection and interpretation in the small bowel, oral contrast should be combined with intravenous contrast material. In most cases we use a very common CT technique that is not dedicated to the detection of peritoneal metastases but dedicated to the metastatic work-up. For CT of the liver we utilize the VENOUS PHASE with images obtained between 70-90 seconds after the injection of contrast Figure 1.5 (top). This recommendation was developed for liver imaging and it is the best timing to see liver metastases. When you perform a work-up optimized for liver metastases, lymphadenopathy, or lung metastases, you should be aware that the CT examination has not been optimized specifically for peritoneal metastases. The problem with the 70-90 second interval is that the contrast of tumor deposits is exactly the same as the contrast of the small bowel or viscera [10].

We can image in the late arterial phase about 30 seconds after the injection of contrast. This timing is preferred in specific cases like hypervascular tumors, NET tumors, or digestive NET tumors associated with peritoneal metastases. We know that in these cases the neuroendocrine deposits often enhance like liver metastases. The middle part of Figure 1.5 is an example of a NET tumor deposit of peritoneal metastases with a high enhancement from late arterial acquisition.

And finally, there is another phase called the enteric phase [11]. This phase is performed 45 seconds after the injection of contrast. This phase is well known to radiologists that perform CT for Crohn's disease because there is better enhancement of the bowel wall. The enteric phase imaging can increase the conspicuity of abnormal small bowel enhancement and mural stratification. The bottom part of Figure 1.5 is an example of high enhancement at the enteric phase of the wall of the small bowel. More often, the jejunal small bowel is more enhanced than the ileum phase. To my knowledge there is no paper or validated data analyzing the value of this phase for peritoneal metastases detection (see Table 1.2).

CT-enteroclysis is an advanced technique described by Courcoutsakis et al, in which they performed CT-enteroclysis to analyze involvement by peritoneal metastases [12]. The goal was to assess specifically small bowel and small bowel mesentery involvement. For the CT-enteroclysis, you need to enforce a very strict technique with fasting 24 hours before the examination, nasojejunal intubation and bowel distension with enteral administration of about 2 liters of polyethylene glycol, as a negative contrast. Then you do a regular CT with intravenous contrast injection. The goal is to obtain small bowel distension to be more likely to see a region of stenosis or distortion. In the manuscript by Courcoutsakis et al., 48 patients eligible for HIPEC had a very high sensitivity and positive predictive value to assess the visceral peritoneum. CT-enteroclysis requires a radiologist dedicated to the study of intestinal imaging as part of the peritoneal malignancy team.

Rather than use CT-enteroclysis our group used a more comfortable CT enterography. Our patients need to fast only 4 hours prior to the examination. There is no need for nasogastric intubation, rather the patient drinks up 1.5 liters of water with methylcellulose or polyethylene glycol over 30 minutes followed by an injection of an antispasmodic agent such as Buscopan (hyoscine butylbromide) (Sanofi, Guildford, Surrey, UK). One can reliably obtain high definition of the small bowel in order to image visceral peritoneal involvement (Figure 1.6).

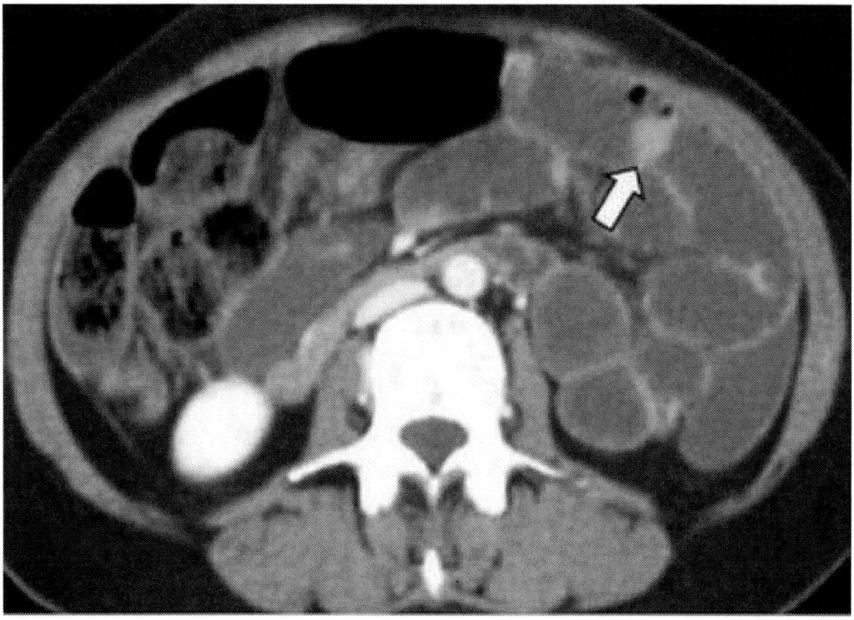

Figure 1.6. CT enterography with positive oral contrast (1.5 liters of water + 45 g of methylcellulose or polyethylene glycol + 70 cc d'accupaque® 300) followed by intravenous injection of 20 mg of Buscopan®. The distension of small-bowel allows a higher conspicuity of the visceral and mesenteric peritoneal implants (arrows).

Table 1.2. Time interval from injection of bolus intravenous contrast to imaging for three separate indications for CT

Phase	Indication	Interval (seconds)
Late arterial	Hypervascular neuroendocrine tumors	30
Enteric	Enhancement of bowel walls	45
Venous	Metastatic disease especially liver metastases	70-90

To summarize thoughts on CT as the reference imaging modality, we need to have standardization of our protocol and a standardization of our CT review. This requires an analysis of the PERITONEUM AS AN ORGAN. I am convinced that this is the main problem of radiologists who are not experts in imaging peritoneal metastases. They look at the liver, spleen, lymph nodes, but they forget to examine specifically the peritoneum. We should, in each case, of colon cancer or ovarian cancer, look at the peritoneum as an organ composed of two parts, the parietal peritoneum and visceral peritoneum. To do this one must use multiplanar reconstruction to increase accuracy. The coronal plane provides better delineation of disease between the liver and the diaphragm. Add time to the review of images for the mesentery. It is more obvious to distinguish between a loop of small bowel and an implant in an axial plane. The sagittal plane is useful to see the greater omentum. If you see that there is an increased thickness of the greater omentum, the probability of cancer infiltration is very high.

We must study not only the intraperitoneal structures but also the peritoneal fat folds because tumor implants develop well in fat. Study the ligaments and mesenteries. We can also see the involvement of the triangular ligament as well as the coronary ligament, falciform ligament, lesser omentum, and the mesentery. Carefully inspect the fat layers in and around the peritoneum (Figure 1.7).

STANDARDIZED REPORTING OF CT

Finally, we have to standardize reporting. We need to use the peritoneal cancer index (PCI) to assess the extent and the distribution of the disease [13]. We can estimate this assessment on CT. There is now some software that allows standardization within multidisciplinary teams and centers. Personally, I use a free internet application called the PROMISE [14]. You are able to systematically analyze CT, MRI, and PET-CT. Also, we are able to add several anatomic regions to the peritoneal cancer index. It is very important to enumerate the organs at risk for disease calling attention to small bowel involvement, the mesenteries, and the lesser omentum. Finally, the computer generates an automatic portable document format (PDF) report so you can place it in the medical records. Or, if you want to perform research you can produce an Excel database.

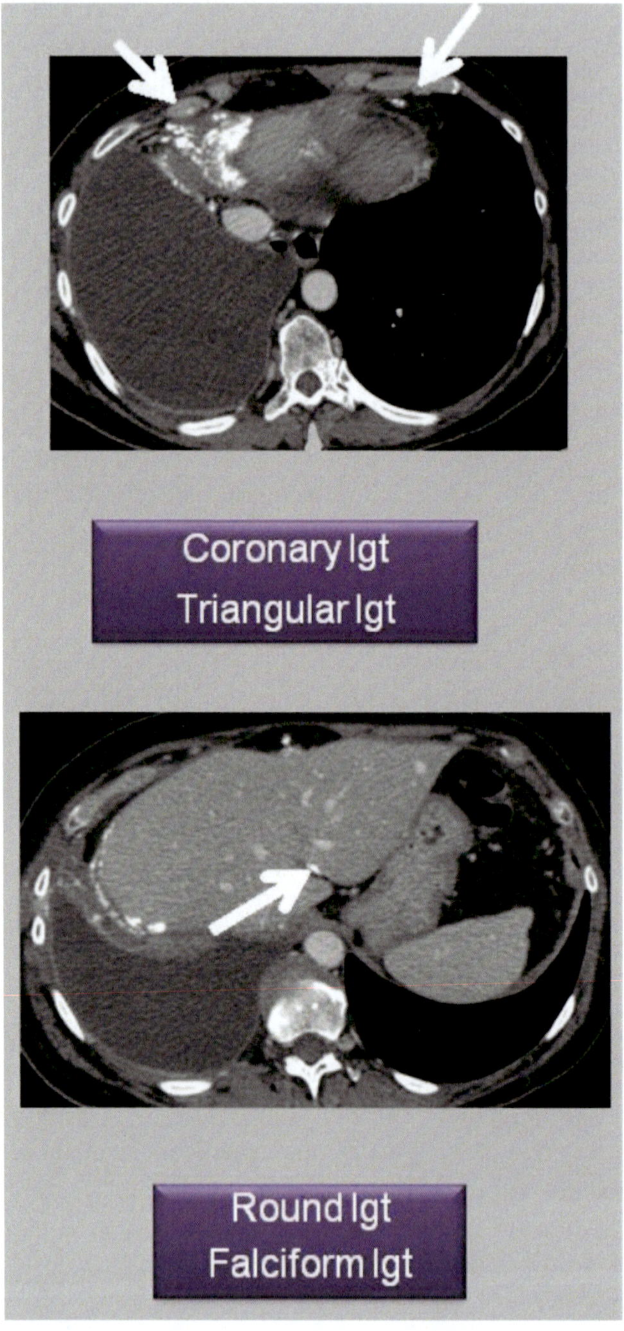

Figure 1.7. (Continued)

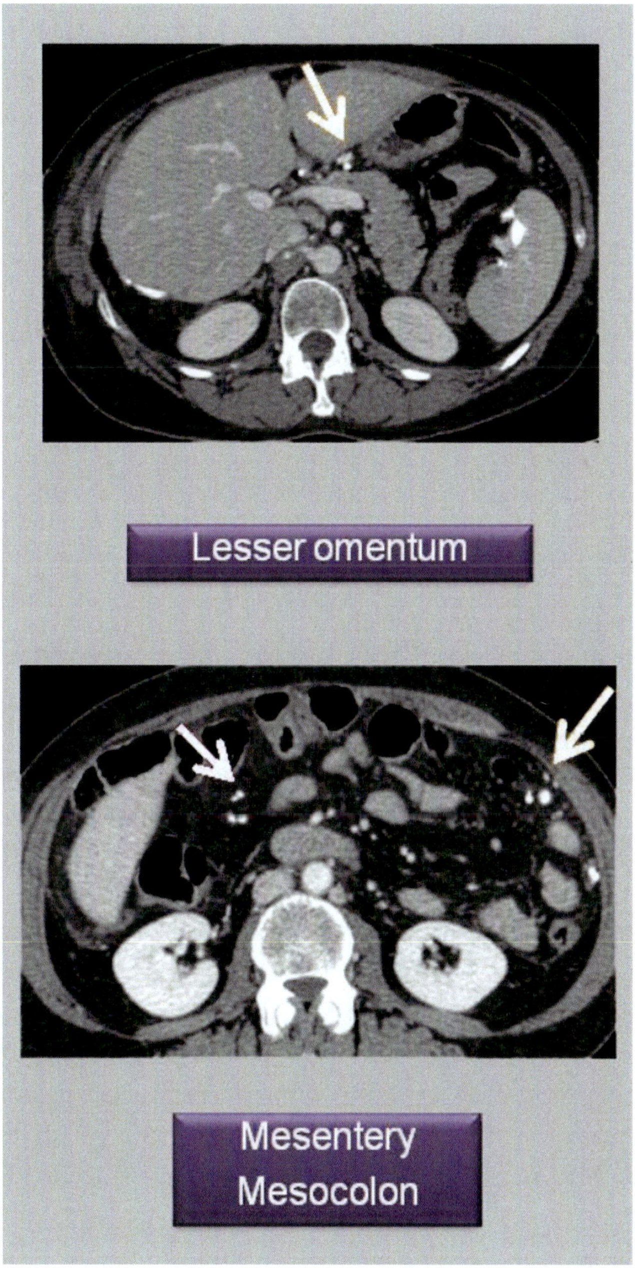

Figure 1.7. Calcified peritoneal metastases from an ovarian psammomacarcinoma. Axial CT images show peritoneal implants in hepatic ligament, lesser omentum and mesentery of the mesocolon (lgt = ligament).

MRI as an Imaging Modality

The next task is to describe the best technology for MRI, including diffusion-weighted imaging. Diffusion-weighted MRI is helpful like PET-CT. It directs the radiologist's attention on review of morphological MRI images to areas of suspected tumor. Diffusion-weighted MRI can increase the contrast of tumor nodules and then we can look retrospectively at morphological images such as T2 or T1 to confirm or deny if there is a tumor implant. MRI of the peritoneum is probably the most difficult MRI we are asked to perform for gastrointestinal cancer. This is because there are a lot of artifacts. Motion artifacts are due to bulk physiologic motions like peristalsis, respiration, and blood flow. There are also susceptibility artifacts found at the lung bases and adjacent to the air-filled segments of bowel which result in geometric distortion. We also have problems with "T2 shine-through effect" which is an area of high intensity. T2 can appear very bright in diffusion-weighted images. This is not due to a restriction effect but due to the high signal intensity. Finally, we have some normal high signal organs in diffusion-weighted images such as the spleen, lymph nodes and adrenal glands. It is really important that diffusion-weighted images should not be performed alone but always in association with morphological imaging. In the absence of morphological imaging, artifacts lead to false negative results and "T2 shine-through effect." Normal high signal can result in false positive results.

The clinical value of MRI is to obtain higher contrast. Some sites have combined gadolinium-enhanced MRI with diffusion-weighted MRI, both of which can increase tumor contrast and conspicuity. Figure 1.8 (top) is a CT examination that shows peritoneal metastases beneath the right hemidiaphragm and within the greater omentum. With the diffusion-weighted MRI the cancer shows greater contrast (Figure 1.8 middle and bottom).

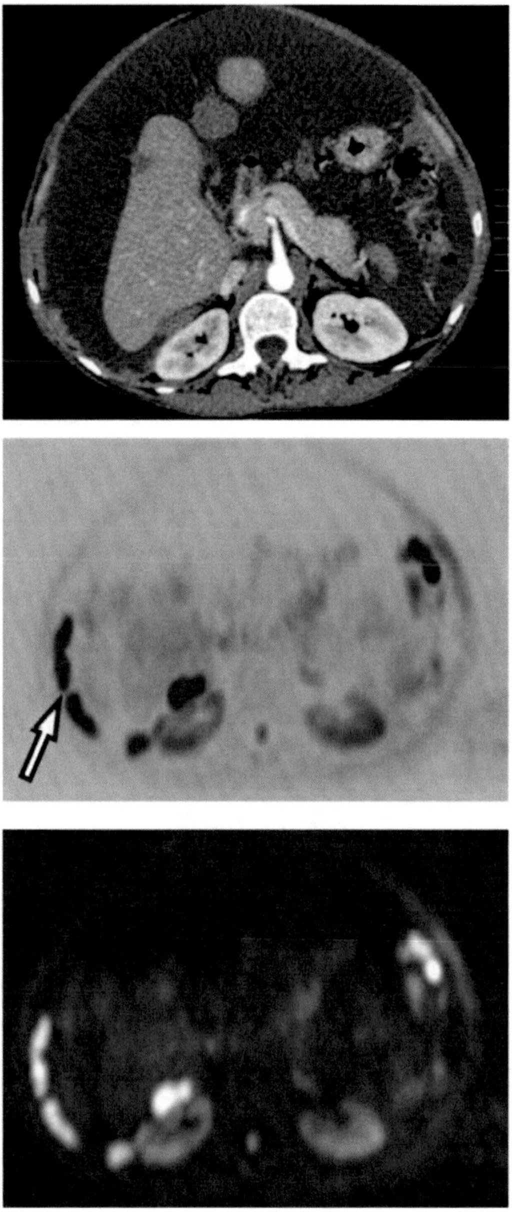

Figure 1.8. Patient with peritoneal metastases from an ovarian cancer. CT image (top) shows a large amount of perihepatic ascites. Diffusion-weighted (middle) and diffusion-weighted with inverted grey white scale (bottom) MRI images increase the conspicuity of peritoneal implants of the parietal peritoneum. Morrisson's pouch and left paracolic gutter were depicted on CT in retrospect.

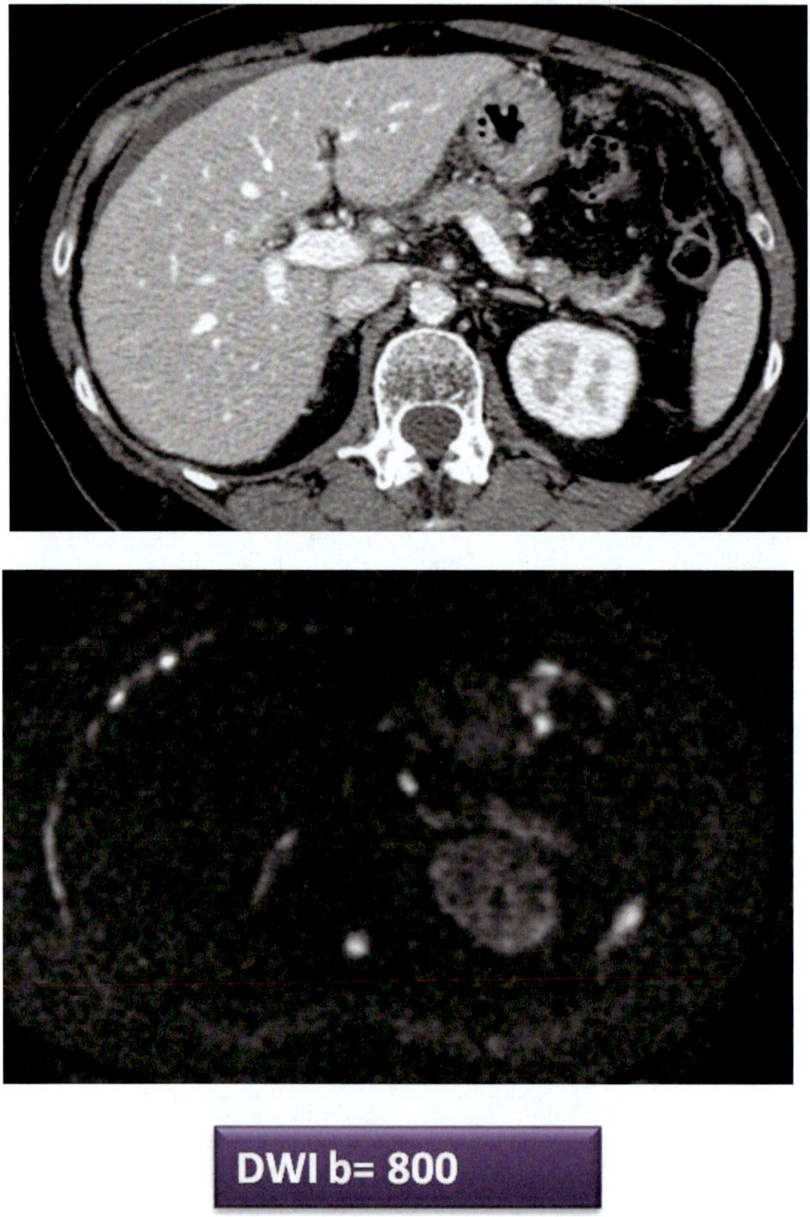

Figure 1.9. (top and bottom). Peritoneal metastases from a colon cancer. CT image (top) show a perihepatic ascites. Diffusion-weighted image (bottom) using high b-value (800) increases the conspicuity of the perihepatic peritoneal implant by the suppression of the signal intensity of ascites fluid.

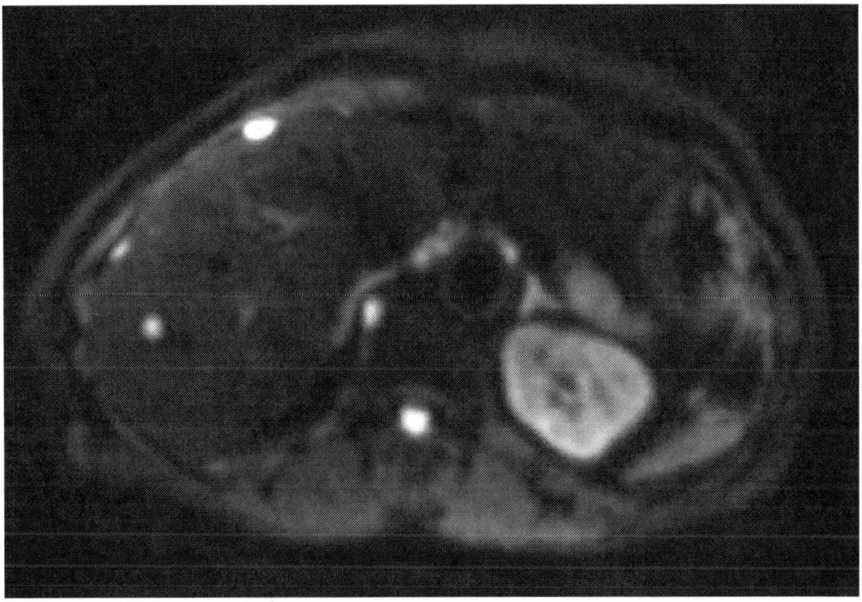

Figure 1.10. Peritoneal metastases from a neuroendocrine tumor. Diffusion-weighted image well depicted with a very high contrast resolution of the multiple perihepatic peritoneal implants.

The high b value increases the conspicuity of some tumoral implants but also there is a suppression of the signal intensity of ascites fluid, fat and small bowel fluid. There is always a compromise because the high b value increases specificity but decreases sensitivity so you have to balance this depending on your scan. This technique is highly sensitive for some anatomic sites such as the perihepatic area and the pelvis and is very accurate in association with T2-weighted images for mucinous pseudomyxoma. For me this is the reference method that we use for pseudomyxoma and mucinous tumors.

Figure 1.9 provides an example of a patient with perihepatic ascites. In these cases it is often difficult to be sure that this is peritoneal metastases and not just fluid. In Figure 1.9 (top), on CT you can only see free ascites fluid. But if you perform diffusion-weighted images, now you see that there is more than ascites in Figure 1.9 (bottom). There are tumor implants present that were not possible to identify on CT examination.

Figure 1.10 provides an example of metastatic disease from a neuroendocrine tumor. We use T2-weighted images and contrast-enhanced images. You can see that the deposits are very bright with diffusion-weighted MRI. There are deposits in the liver and involvement of the lesser omentum. You can easily make a complete assessment.

Standardized Reporting of MRI

In France, there is a standardized protocol for MRI because not all radiologists are very familiar with the technique that we are using. You probably know the RENAPE group for surgeons. We have a subgroup for radiologists known as RENA-RAD. We published a common protocol for the surgeons to give to their patients before they have their MRI examination. First, preparation is crucial to reduce bowel motion artifacts. The patient is asked to fast at least 6 hours prior the examination. Also to reduce peristalsis, an intravenous injection of Glucagon (Eli Lilly and Company, Indianapolis, IN) or Buscopan (hyoscine butylbromide, Sanofi, Guilford, Surrey, UK) before and during the MRI by slow infusion. The mandatory sequences are as follow: Diffusion-weighted images with a b value greater than or equal to 800 s/mm^2, T2-weighted without fat suppression, T1-weighted after contrast in the axial and frontal plan 3-5 minutes after the injection of contrast. Optional sequences include: Fat suppression by single-shot fast spin-echo (SSFSE) – this is very useful if you have pseudomyxoma or mucinous tumor. If you are looking for pseudocystic lesions, you really need to be able to increase the contrast. You can also perform dynamic T1-weighted images particularly in the liver or in the abdomen to rule out liver metastases in patients with colon cancer.

Figure 1.11 presents a case of recurrent pseudomyxoma. This is the CT examination below and the diffusion-weighted MRI images above. You can see that it is much easier by MRI to detect the very small area of recurrent mucinous tumor. You can also see well by MRI the involvement of the seminal vesicle. By CT it is very difficult to be sure that this is tumor and not normal anatomy. On MRI you can clearly see a tumor deposit. Retrospectively, once again you see with the help of MRI all the deposits on the CT examination so you are sure this is not an artifact.

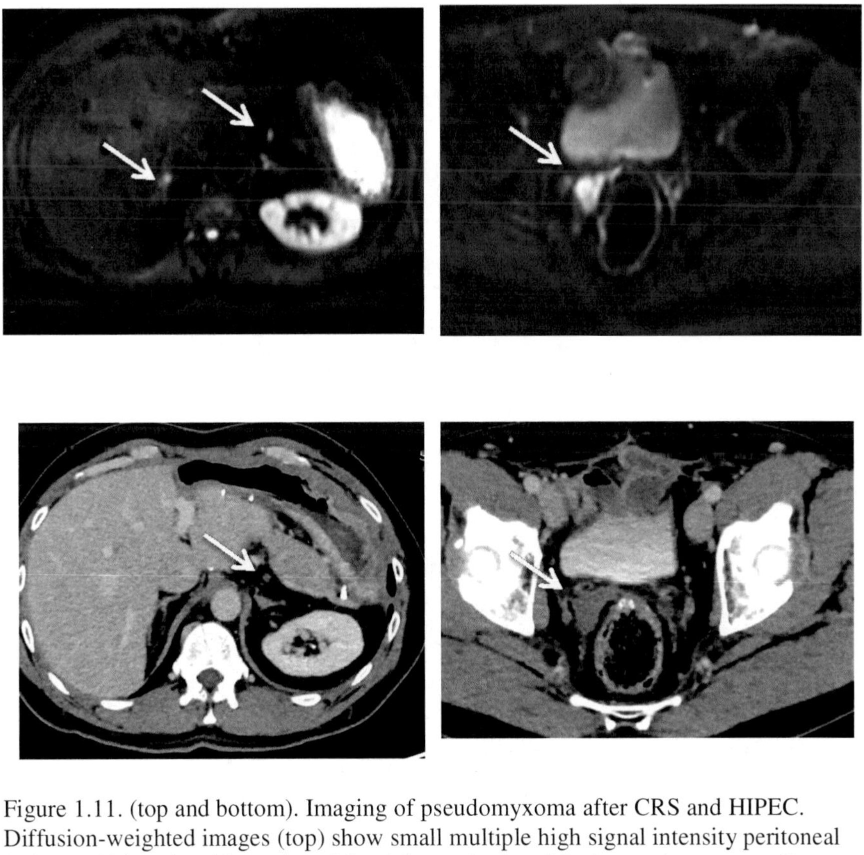

Figure 1.11. (top and bottom). Imaging of pseudomyxoma after CRS and HIPEC. Diffusion-weighted images (top) show small multiple high signal intensity peritoneal lesion and high signal intensity of the right seminal vesicle (arrows) corresponding to recurrent peritoneal implants. These implants are more difficult to detect on CT images due to their lower contrast (bottom).

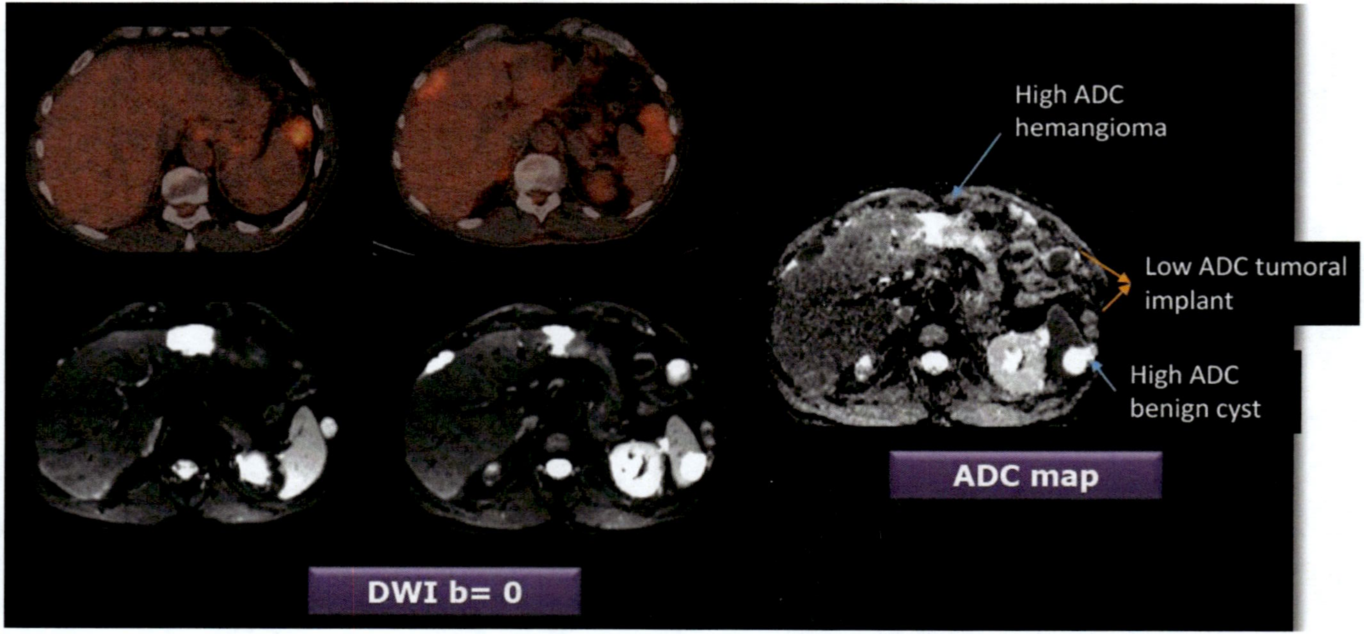

Figure 1.12. (top and bottom). Imaging of hepatic hemangioma and peritoneal metastases. FDG-PET-CT images (top) show 3 peritoneal lesions with high tracer uptake. On MRI images (bottom), benign and malignant lesions could have similar appearance with high signal intensity on T2-weighted images and low b value diffusion-weighted sequence. ADC map is required to distinguish benign lesion with high signal intensity from malignant lesion with low signal intensity.

To overcome the problem of T2 shine through, you can consult the apparent diffusion coefficient map (ADC map). For this reason we always perform two b values. As an example, in Figure 1.12 we have by MRI, very intense areas. If we look at the ADC map the omental lesions have a low ADC corresponding to a tumoral implant. Whereas on the ADC map the liver lesion was a hemangioma and the other a very common cystic spleen lesion. This clarification of T2 shine through is the task of the radiologist and we have the tools to be able to distinguish benign from malignant lesions.

PET-CT as an Imaging Modality

To finish up our standardization of best technology, a brief presentation of PET-CT is necessary. It is similar to diffusion-weighted MRI. The PET has high contrast of nodules and it enables the visualization of peritoneal implants retrospectively seen but not recognized as peritoneal metastases on CT. It can be of value in some locations that are very difficult to image on CT such as small bowel, mesentery, and pelvis. And, it has a high inter-reader reproducibility. A recent meta-analysis by Li et al. found a 84% sensitivity and 98% specificity for PET-CT [15]. This is not the case for CT and MRI, but for PET-CT it is an advantage. Figure 1.13 is an example of tumor that is well detected on PET-CT. Retrospectively you can often see the lesion on CT, but you are more confident since this area lights up well on PET-CT. Although CT and PET-CT complement each other, in most studies the per-site analysis by PET-CT is not superior to CT. Also, both PET-CT and CT significantly underestimate the number of regions involved by tumor. The two modalities used together increase diagnostic accuracy.

Finally, PET-CT can facilitate the selection of patients suitable for cytoreductive surgery by ruling out extraperitoneal disease. Sometimes we have atypical mediastinal lymph node metastases, or subclavicular lymph node metastases that are not depicted at all with CT or MRI. PET-CT is important if you expect extraperitoneal disease.

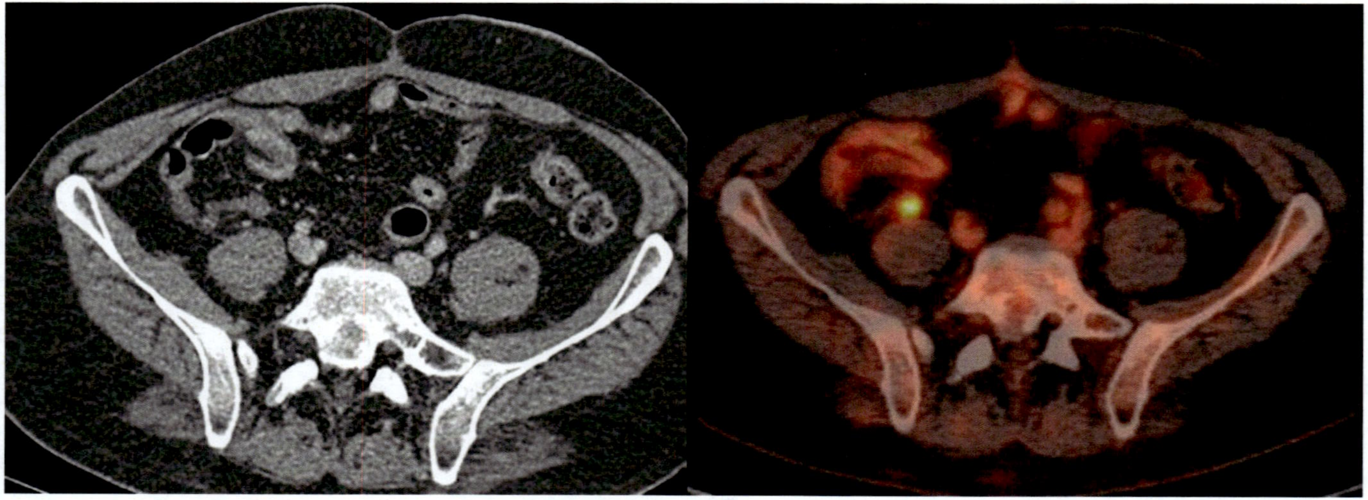

Figure 1.13. (left and right). Peritoneal metastases from a colon cancer. On CT images (left) peritoneal metastases, even if large in size, are difficult to distinguish from the normal small bowel. FDG-PET-CT images (right) increase the detectability of peritoneal metastases due to the high contrast of lesions. Note that most lesions detected on PET-CT are retrospectively seen on CT images, although they are isodense to normal anatomy.

FUTURE PROSPECTS FOR PET

The detection of peritoneal metastases with PET-CT will provide increasing benefit due to recent advances with PET-CT technology. We say that tumor implants less than 1 cm in diameter are not detected by PET-CT. Probably that will change because the technology is constantly improving. We have reduced acquisition time with new PET-CT technology. That could result in reduced false negative interpretations due to small bowel motion. We have higher detector sensitivity and the ability to detect small amount of tracer uptake. We have the time of flight (TOF) technology with fast scintillating material and fast photon detectors that allows an increase spatial resolution from 1 cm to 5 mm. Finally, an increased reproducibility of standardized uptake values (SUV) quantification. As a result of this progress, in the future the results will be better in the detection of peritoneal metastases. We also know that there are newer tracers. Actually, we use FDG in most cases, particularly for colon cancer but the tracer must be adapted to the tumor type and we can use F-DOPA for digestive well-differentiated neuroendocrine tumors (WD NET) tumors, Ga-DOTATOC in other WD NET tumors, F-Fluorocholine for WD hepatocellular (HCC), and so on.

To conclude, the optimization and standardization of imaging technology is crucial for peritoneal metastases detection and selection of patients suitable for cytoreductive surgery and perioperative chemotherapy. Improved imaging technology will also facilitate multicenter clinical trials and longitudinal studies of response to therapy. However, with peritoneal metastases, technology alone is not enough! The technology is important but accurate interpretation will significantly improve the per-site detection of peritoneal metastases.

References

[1] Sugarbaker PH, Sardi A, Brown G, Dromain C, Rousset P, Jelinek JS. Concerning CT features used to select patients for treatment of peritoneal metastases, a pictoral essay. *Int J Hyperthermia*. 2017;33(5):497-504.

[2] Dromain C, Leboulleux S, Auperin A, Goere D, Malka D, Lumbroso J, Schumberger M, Sigal R, Elias D. Staging of peritoneal carcinomatosis: enhanced CT vs. PET/CT. *Abdom Imaging*. 2008;33(1):87-93.

[3] Jacquet P, Jelinek JS, Steves MA, Sugarbaker PH. Evaluation of computed tomography in patients with peritoneal carcinomatosis. *Cancer*. 1993;72(5):1631-6.

[4] Davies J, Chalmers AG, Sue-Ling HM, May J, Miller GV, Martin IG, Johnston D. Spiral computed tomography and operative staging of gastric carcinoma: a comparison with histopathological staging. *Gut*. 1997;41(3):314-9.

[5] de Bree E, Koops W, Kröger R, van Ruth S, Witkamp AJ, Zoetmulder FA. Peritoneal carcinomatosis from colorectal or appendiceal origin: correlation of preoperative CT with intraoperative findings and evaluation of interobserver agreement. *J Surg Oncol*. 2004;86(2):64-73.

[6] Koh DM, Blackledge M, Collins DJ, Padhani AR, Wallace T, Wilton B, Taylor NJ, Stirling JJ, Sinha R, Walicke P, Leach MO, Judson I, Nathan P. Reproducibility and changes in the apparent diffusion coefficients of solid tumours treated with combretastatin A4 phosphate and bevacizumab in a two-centre phase I clinical trial. *Eur Radiol*. 2009;19(11):2728-38.

[7] Kim SJ, Kim HH, Kim YH, Hwang SH, Lee HS, Park DJ, Kim SY, Lee KH. Peritoneal metastasis: detection with 16- or 64-detector row CT in patients undergoing surgery for gastric cancer. *Radiology*. 2009;253(2):407-15.

[8] Marin D, Catalano C, Baski M, Di Martino M, Geiger D, Di Giorgio A, Sibio S, Passariello R. 64-Section multi-detector row CT in the

preoperative diagnosis of peritoneal carcinomatosis: correlation with histopathological findings. *Abdom Imaging*. 2010;35(6):694-700.

[9] Warde P, Rideout DF, Herman S, Majesky IF, Sturgeon JF, Fine S, Boyd NF. Computed tomography in advanced ovarian cancer: an evaluation of diagnostic accuracy. *Am J Med Sci*. 1987;293(2):94-8.

[10] Coakley FV, Choi PH, Gougoutas CA, Pothuri B, Venkatraman E, Chi D, Bergman A, Hricak H. Peritoneal metastases: detection with spiral CT in patients with ovarian cancer. *Radiology*. 2002;223(2):495-9.

[11] Booya F, Fletcher JG, Huprich JE, Barlow JM, Johnson CD, Fidler JL, Solem CA, Sandborn WJ, Loftus EV Jr, Harmsen WS. Active Crohn disease: CT findings and interobserver agreement for enteric phase CT enterography. *Radiology*. 2006;241(3):787-95.

[12] Courcoutsakis N, Tentes AA, Astrinakis E, Zezos P, Prassopoulos P. CT-Enteroclysis in the preoperative assessment of the small-bowel involvement in patients with peritoneal carcinomatosis, candidates for cytoreductive surgery and hyperthermic intraperitoneal chemotherapy. *Abdom Imaging*. 2013;38(1):56-63.

[13] Jacquet P, Sugarbaker PH. Current methodologies for clinical assessment of patients with peritoneal carcinomatosis. *J Exp Clin Cancer Res*. 1996;15(1):49-58.

[14] *PROMISE* (PeRitOneal MalIgnancy Stage Evaluation) Internet Application accessed at http://www.e-promise.org/.

[15] Li J, Yan R, Lei J, Jiang C. Comparison of PET with PET/CT in detecting peritoneal carcinomatosis: a meta-analysis. *Abdom Imaging*. 2015;40(7):2660-6.

In: Pictorial Essays … ISBN: 978-1-53618-014-5
Editors: PH Sugarbaker and RN Low ©2020 Nova Science Publishers, Inc.

Chapter 2

Formulating a Lexicon of Concerning Radiologic Features for Peritoneal Metastases

James S. Jelinek, MD, FACR
Department of Radiology, MedStar Washington Hospital Center, Washington, DC, US

Introduction

The natural history of gastrointestinal and gynecologic malignancy often results in cancer dissemination to the peritoneal surfaces of the abdomen and pelvis. In the past such dissemination was referred to as peritoneal carcinomatosis but more recently it is referred to as peritoneal metastases. A successful treatment strategy for peritoneal metastases involves cytoreductive surgery (CRS) combined with hyperthermic intraperitoneal chemotherapy (HIPEC) [1]. This combination of treatments has been accepted for treatment of selected patients in most countries in Europe and in the United States [2, 3]. All centers reporting their data regarding CRS and HIPEC agree that complete surgical resection is an absolute requirement for long-term benefit of the combined treatment (4).

To facilitate the likelihood of successful complete surgical resection, knowledgeable preoperative patient selection is mandatory. This manuscript describes important prognostic information that can be gleaned from a technically optimized pretreatment CT scan. Concerning CT features that might preclude complete surgical cytoreduction are described in detail.

The concerning CT features depicted on a pretreatment CT identifies a condition(s) that makes complete CRS more difficult or impossible. Also, it identifies patients whose CRS will require added complexity so that the morbidity and mortality of the surgical intervention will be increased. The goal for this presentation is to provide a lexicon of concerning radiologic features for peritoneal metastases. This is an attempt to name them, describe the radiologic appearance on CT, and then suggest their utility in the surgical management of peritoneal metastases. The list may not be complete as more subtle radiologic techniques such as diffusion-weighted MRI and PET-CT are used knowledgeably for the many different malignancies that disseminate within the peritoneal spaces. Currently, 15 concerning CT features from pretreatment CT are identified to assist in the management of peritoneal metastases patients.

Principles of Peritoneal Metastases Dissemination Important to the Radiologist

Tumor Histology

Before the concerning CT features are described some principles that guide the utilization of these images may be helpful. First, data from long-term follow-up has firmly established that tumor grade, invasive malignant versus non-invasive, makes a large difference in outcome in the use of CRS and HIPEC. These tumor types include pseudomyxoma peritonei and appendiceal tumors, low malignant potential ovarian tumors and ovarian cancers, colorectal, and gastric malignancy. Both low grade and high-grade peritoneal mesotheliomas are included. For all of these tumor types a complete cytoreduction is going to be the only resection to eventuate in 5-year survival. The histology of the specific neoplasm must be combined with the CT features to estimate which patient are likely to undergo a complete versus an incomplete cytoreduction. Tumor histology in combination with recognition of concerning radiologic features functions as an important selection tool in peritoneal metastases patients.

Parietal versus Visceral Peritoneum

Second, there is a large difference in the surgeons' capacity to completely resect tumor nodules associated with parietal peritoneum as compared to visceral peritoneum. The peritonectomy procedures are, with a few exceptions, a stripping of parietal peritoneum. High-voltage ball tip electrosurgery allows, if necessary, a complete resection of all parietal peritoneum including that from beneath right and left hemidiaphragms, the right and left paracolic sulci, the retroperitoneum, the pelvis and the posterior aspect of the omental bursa [5].

In sharp contrast, nodules on visceral peritoneum may preclude complete cytoreduction. There is a well-defined limit to possible resections of stomach, small bowel, and colorectum. Most frequently the cancer nodules that limit the possibility of a complete cytoreduction are located on visceral peritoneum of the small bowel or its mesentery. Invasive peritoneal cancer nodules on small bowel or large bowel surface or mesentery routinely require resection of the involved structure. Occasionally, if mesenteric invasion and retraction are limited, resections of peritoneum at the base of small or large bowel mesentery are possible [6]. However, cancer nodules at the junction of small bowel with its mesentery require segmental small bowel resection [5]. Also, cancer invading along the lesser curvature of the stomach and involving the vascular arcade of the right and left gastric arteries may not be resectable unless a near total gastrectomy can be tolerated by the patient. It is not only the extent of peritoneal metastases but their location that may determine the possibility of complete resection.

Peritoneum as a First Line of Defense

To summarize, parietal peritonectomy is effective in complete resection of the cancerous implants at a majority of anatomic sites; while visceral peritoneal implants present a much greater challenge for complete cytoreduction. Finally, realizing that the peritoneum is the first line of defense against abdominal and pelvic dissemination, the extent of prior surgery may be an important factor determining complete versus incomplete cytoreduction [7]. The capacity of cancerous implants to penetrate through intact peritoneum is limited. For a limited time period the nodules are contained by the peritoneum without evidence of invasion beneath the connective tissue layer. Cancer cells implanting at sites of disrupted peritoneal surfaces are invasive from the time of first progression.

A site for failure of peritoneal defenses against carcinomatosis is a disrupted peritoneal surface that occurs naturally within the abdomen and pelvis. The Krukenberg tumor is a natural demonstration of tumor cell entrapment [8]. Free cancer cells in the peritoneal cavity from a gastrointestinal cancer adhere to the raw surface created by the corpus hemorrhagicum. Ovarian metastases are frequently the first manifestation of peritoneal dissemination in the female patient.

Perhaps the most common disruption of the peritoneal barrier to cancer cells occurs as a result of surgical dissection. This can be expected in any patient who has undergone abdominal or pelvic surgery in the presence of free intraperitoneal neoplastic cells. For example, trocar site recurrence after laparoscopic biopsy of patients with diffuse malignant peritoneal mesothelioma frequently occurs. Also, ovarian cancer recurrence within the vaginal cuff post-hysterectomy is a common site for cancer progression requiring additional surgery. Another common site for recurrent ovarian cancer is the lower aspect of the abdominal incision. It is the cause of suture line recurrence in patients with a rectal cancer and low colorectal anastomosis. Sometimes these cancer cells come from within the lumen of the colorectum; more frequently cancer cells are present within the pelvis and become entrapped at the anastomotic site or within the raw tissue created by the rectal resection. Of course, if extensive peritonectomy is performed with peritoneal metastases present, a broad layering of cancer deep to the peritoneal surface may result. These patients become untreatable by subsequent peritonectomy procedures and are poor candidates for CRS and HIPEC.

Fifteen Concerning Radiologic Features

Table 2.1. Fifteen concerning radiologic features observed on preoperative CT as a prognostic assessment for patients with peritoneal metastases

• *Concerning features associated with images of small bowel and its mesentery*
Bowel obstruction or partial obstruction at more than 1 site (Figure 2.1)
Mesentery drawn together by tumor (Figure 2.2)
Tumor infiltrating between leaves of small bowel mesentery (Figure 2.3)
Tumor ≥ 5 cm in diameter in jejunal regions (Figure 2.4)
CT-peritoneal cancer index > 20 [excluding pseudomyxoma peritonei, cystic mesothelioma or low malignant potential ovarian tumors] (Figure 2.6)
• *Concerning features associated with the retroperitoneum*
Mesenteric or para-aortic lymphadenopathy (Figure 2.7)
Hydroureter (Figure 2.8)
Psoas muscle invasion (Figure 2.9)
• *Concerning features associated with pelvic images*
Pelvic sidewall invasion (Figure 2.10)
Seminal vesicle invasion (Figures 2.11A and 2.11B)
• *Concerning features associated with gastrohepatic or hepatoduodenal ligaments*
Porta hepatis infiltration and/or bile duct obstruction
Tumor ≥ 5 cm in diameter in gastrohepatic ligament or subpyloric space (Figure 2.12)
Gastric outlet obstruction (Figure 2.13)
• *Concerning features associated with ascites*
Hemorrhagic ascites
Serous ascites in a gastrointestinal cancer patient (Figure 2.14)

Table 2.1 lists the concerning radiologic features, which may be evaluated on the preoperative CT by the radiologist, who is a member of the multidisciplinary team. These features offer a prognostic assessment of the likelihood of complete cytoreduction. These 15 concerning radiologic features are divided into five categories that include images of small bowel and its mesentery, retroperitoneal images, pelvic images, gastrohepatic or hepatoduodenal ligaments images, and images associated with ascites [9].

Concerning Radiologic Features Associated with Images of Small Bowel and Its Mesentery

Figure 2.1 presents a CT slice through the mid-abdomen that shows loops of small bowel obstructed or partially obstructed at more than one site. The loops of bowel lack uniformity in their diameter and are irregular in their shape.

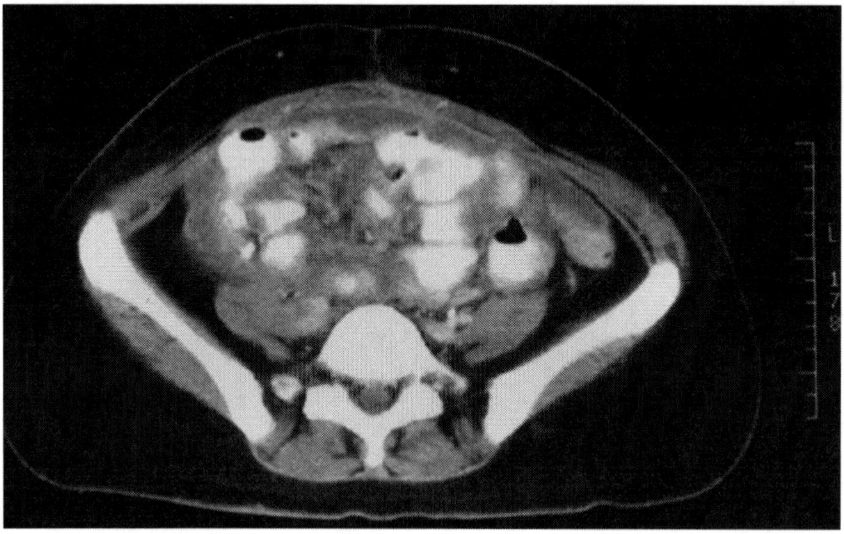

Figure 2.1. CT slice showing bowel obstruction or partial obstruction at more than one site (chaotic bowel pattern).

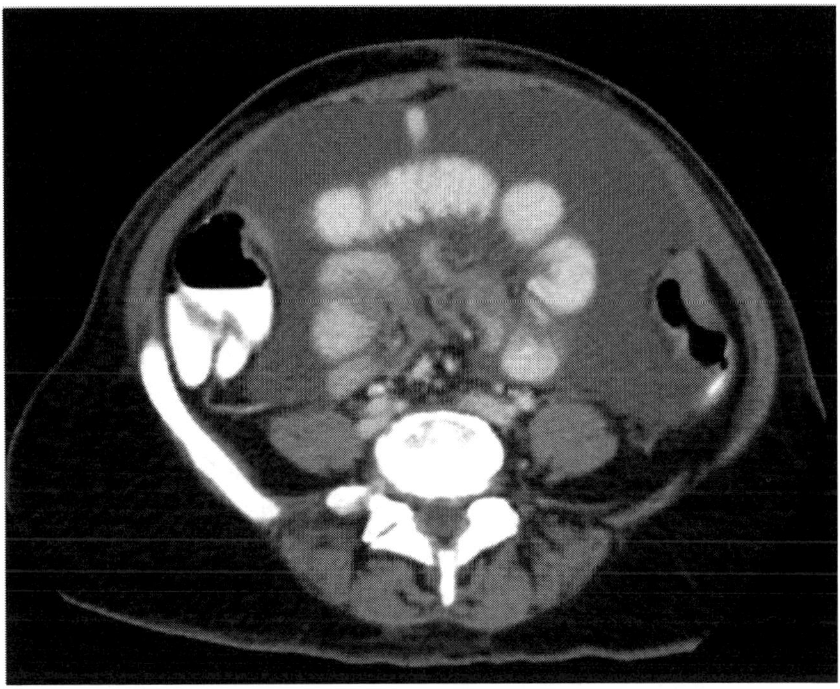

Figure 2.2. CT slice showing mesentery drawn together by tumor (clumped bowel).

The wall of the bowel loops are thickened suggesting a layering of cancer is present. There is fat stranding of the adjacent small bowel mesentery. Multiple loops are irregular suggesting multiple sites of partial obstruction. If the patient had prior surgery, intestinal adhesions may be infiltrated by cancer. The complete cytoreduction of invasive disease on small bowel or small bowel mesentery is usually limited to small bowel resection. Sometimes several segments of bowel with cancerous nodules can be resected so that a major portion of functional small bowel is spared. Unfortunately, cancerous nodules distributed along the small bowel are a prominent cause of incomplete cytoreduction.

Figure 2.2 is a CT slice showing the mesentery clumped together by tumor. This is a strong predictor of diffuse involvement of visceral peritoneum by a tumor of high grade histology. The small bowel itself may appear relatively normal with the mesentery foreshortened toward the retroperitoneum. The cause is a layering of sclerotic cancer on the surface of the small bowel mesentery. The leaves of the mesentery may be fused together. A fibrous contraction of the mesentery and bowel toward the retroperitoneum causes the clumped appearance. The complete cytoreduction of clumped small bowel mesentery is not usually possible. This radiologic image is usually considered an absolute contraindication to any attempt at complete cytoreduction.

Figure 2.3 is a CT slice showing spaces between leaves of the mesentery separated from each other by tumor nodules. The separation is not caused by ascites fluid. The tissue between the leaves of mesentery may, in some cases, appear as a layer but, in other areas nodules are present. The bowel is usually not obstructed nor is the mesentery foreshortened. If the malignancy is of large volume, mucinous, and of low-grade histology this separation of the leaves of the mesentery may not prevent resection of tumor. Knowing the histologic type is important.

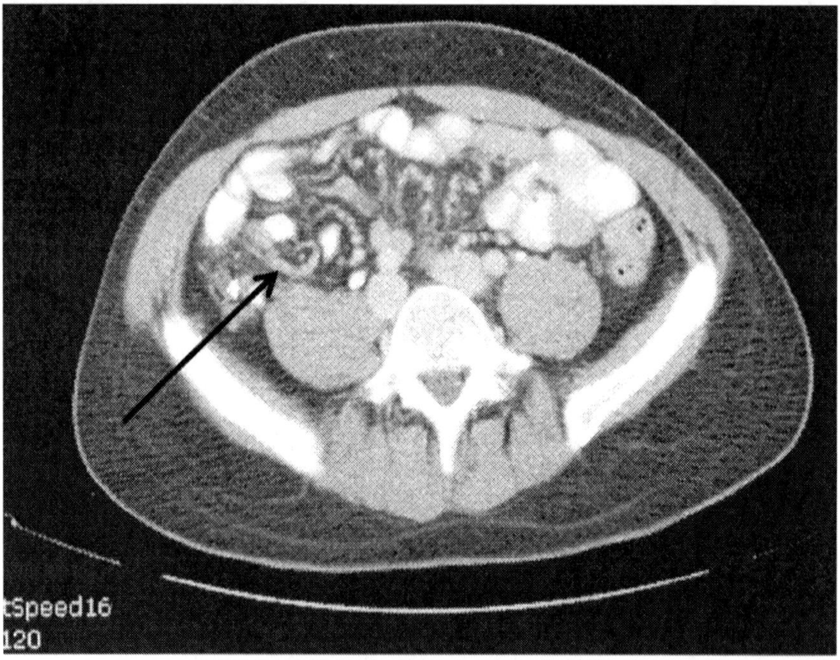

Figure 2.3. CT slice showing tumor infiltrating between leaves of small bowel mesentery (string of pearls).

The anatomic pathology is a continuing accumulation of cancerous nodules which eventually become confluent. As the tumor progresses it causes separation of the leaves of the mesentery and invasion into the visceral peritoneum of the small bowel mesentery. Peritoneal mesothelioma may be a cause of this anatomic pathology. Except in a low-grade malignancy, patients demonstrating separation of the leaves of the mesentery are at greater risk for incomplete cytoreduction. In some patients, especially those with peritoneal mesothelioma, mesenteric peritonectomy may be effective [6]. However, complete resection of invasive small bowel mesenteric tumor is rarely possible.

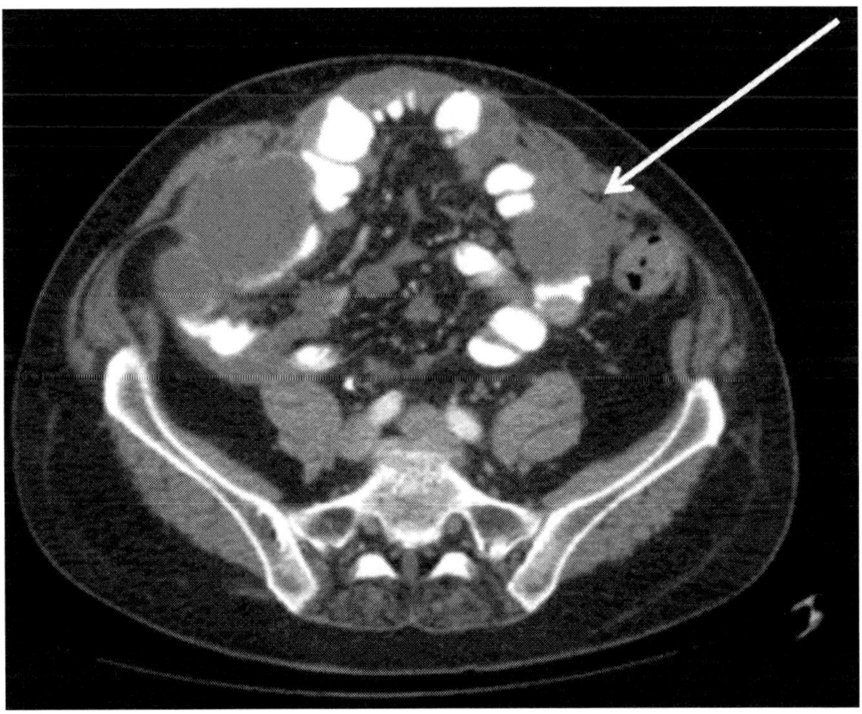

Figure 2.4. CT slice showing tumor ≥ 5 cm in diameter in jejunal regions. There are also large tumor masses present in the ileal regions.

The CT slice in Figure 2.4 shows a tumor nodule greater than 5 cm in diameter on the left side of the mid-abdomen associated with jejunal bowel or bowel mesentery. Extensive involvement of visceral peritoneum of the small bowel and its mesentery, is a common cause for incomplete cytoreduction. There are portions of the small bowel that can be resected if there are tumor nodules present. The small bowel resections that are best tolerated are distal small bowel, especially the terminal part of the ileum. In contrast, resections of proximal small bowel are technically more difficult and are poorly tolerated by the patient from a nutritional perspective. Also, if there are jejunal tumor masses, diffuse small bowel involvement often is present.

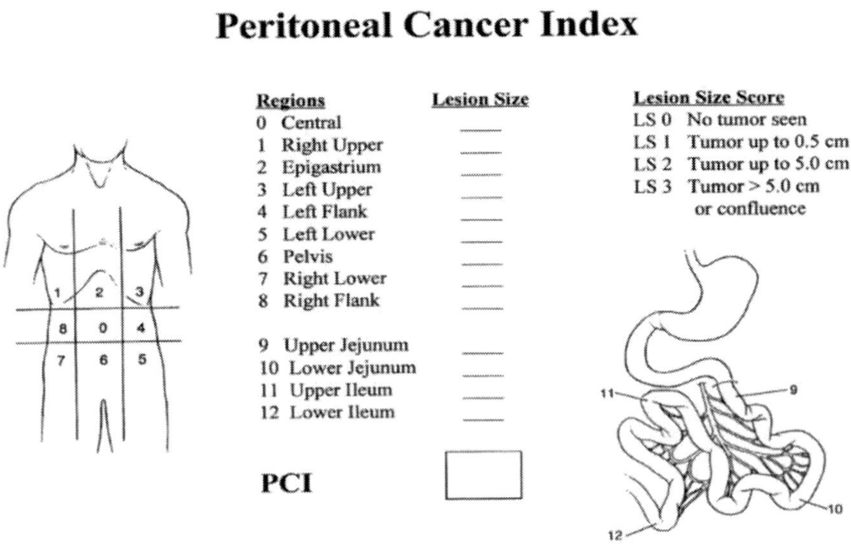

Figure 2.5. The peritoneal cancer index (PCI). The PCI combines size and distribution parameters to determine a numerical score. The lesion size (LS) is used to quantitate the size of peritoneal nodules. LS-0 indicates no tumor seen, LS-1 indicates tumor implants up to 0.5 cm, LS-2 indicates tumor implants between 0.5 and 5 cm, and LS-3 indicates tumor implants larger than 5 cm or a layering of cancer. The distribution of tumor is determined within the 13 abdominopelvic regions. The small bowel is assessed as an additional 4 abdominopelvic regions designated AR-9 through AR-12). (From reference 10 with permission)

An assessment of small bowel involvement by small bowel regions may be helpful for preoperative radiologic predications of complete versus suboptimal cytoreduction [10]. Involvement of peritoneal cancer index regions 9 and 10, the jejunal regions, has more ominous prognostic implications than involvement of regions 11 and 12 (Figure 2.5). The CT-PCI is a global assessment of peritoneal metastases within the abdomen and pelvis [11]. Unfortunately, the failure of CT to demonstrate small tumor nodules limits the utility of CT-PCI for a prognostic assessment of peritoneal metastases [12]. A low CT-PCI does have some prognostic implication, but it will often require revision when the PCI from exploratory laparotomy is determined. In contrast, a high CT-PCI is a reliable prognostic assessment. If the CT depicts tumor nodules, they are almost always present.

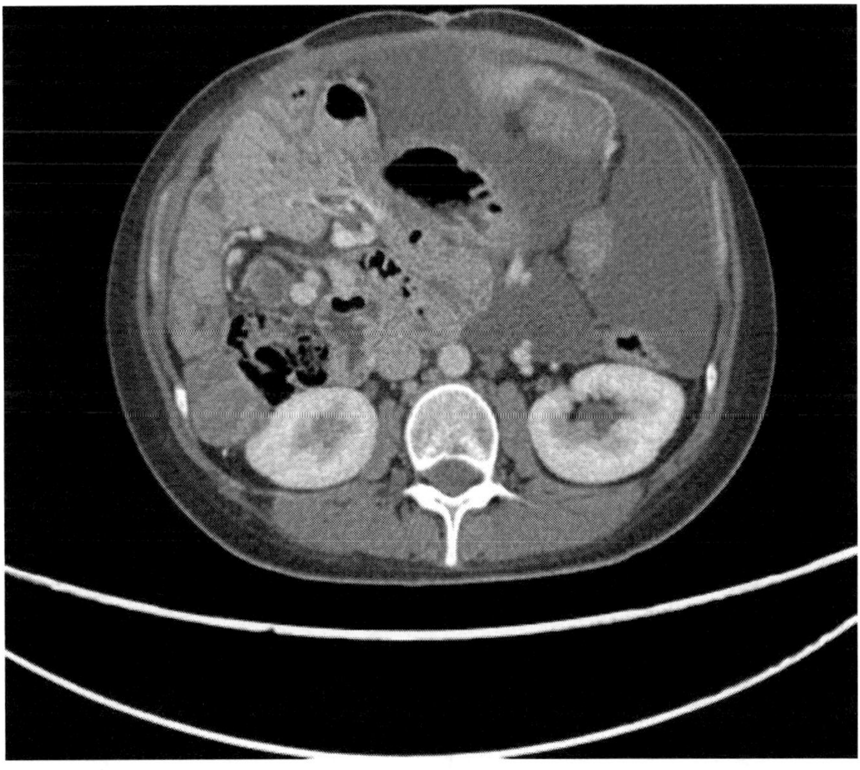

Figure 2.6. CT slice in patient whose CT peritoneal cancer index (PCI) was 24.

For peritoneal metastases from an invasive malignancy, if the CT-PCI is 20 or greater the likelihood of optimal cytoreduction is extremely low. PCI from 0 to 10 may carry a favorable outcome although multiple small tumor nodules may be present and cause an unfavorable outcome. CT-PCI of 10–20 is suggestive but not confirmatory of an unfavorable outcome (Figure 2.6).

These general remarks about CT-PCI require some qualification. CT-PCI accuracy with mucinous tumor is considerably greater than with intestinal type tumor. In general, the more mucinous the malignancy, the more reliable the CT-PCI becomes. With mucinous appendiceal tumors, the CT-PCI becomes quite accurate and can be trusted to provide an accurate radiologic assessment of the extent and anatomic location of pseudomyxoma peritonei [13].

Concerning Radiologic Features Associated with Retroperitoneal Images

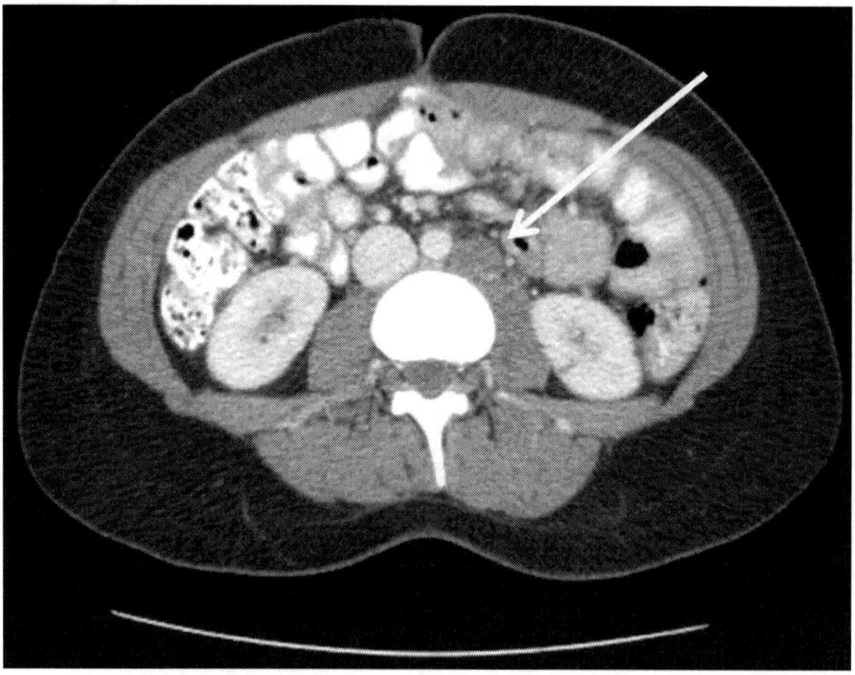

Figure 2.7. CT slice showing para-aortic lymphadenopathy.

If peritoneal metastases are associated with infiltration of the retroperitoneal lymph nodes or structures, the likelihood of a complete cytoreductive surgery is low. Mesenteric and/or para-aortic lymph node infiltration indicates a poor outcome. Complete resection may be difficult because this dissemination indicates high-grade invasive disease that is progressing outside the peritoneal space (Figure 2.7). Retroperitoneal nodularity on CT images may be due to peritoneal metastatic tumor nodules, which can be resected with a clear margin, or may be due to progressive metastatic disease involving lymph nodes. These two different etiologies for retroperitoneal nodularity have very different prognostic implications.

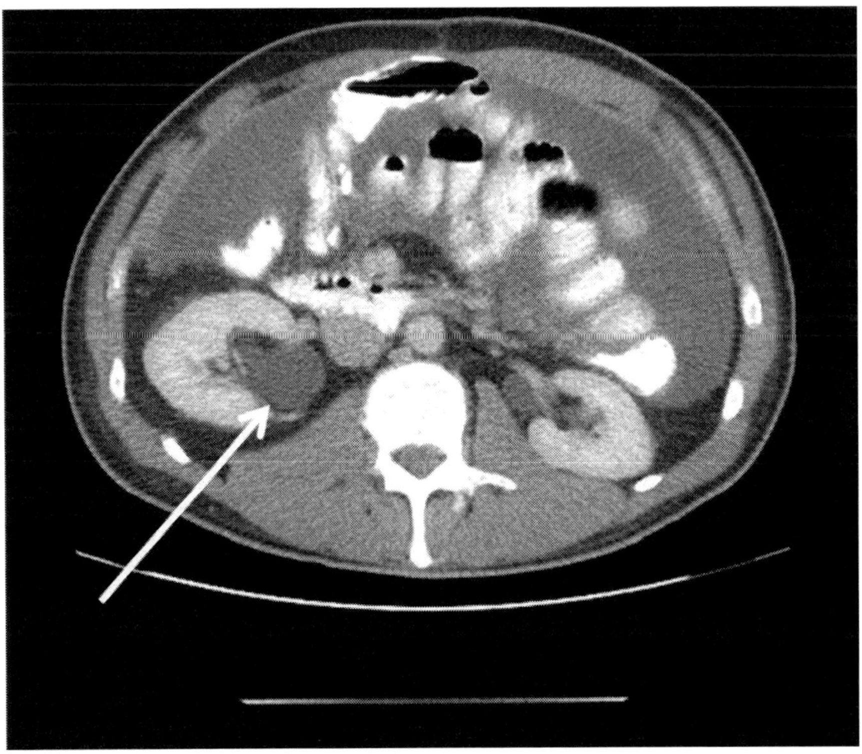

Figure 2.8. CT slice showing right pelvicaliectasis that may be caused by retroperitoneal cancer invasion of the right ureter.

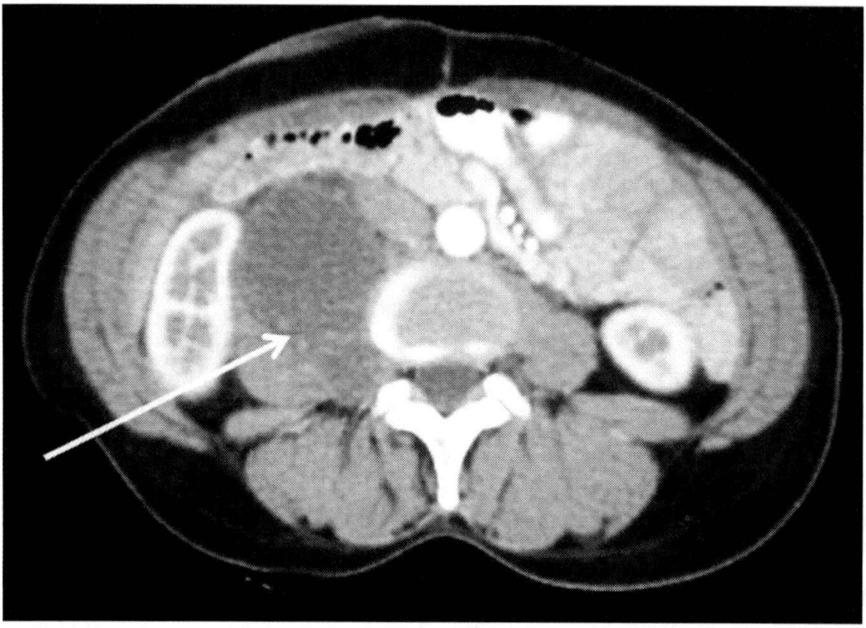

Figure 2.9. CT slice showing psoas muscle invasion. The mucinous appendiceal adenocarcinoma invaded extensively along the psoas muscle.

A CT finding that is associated with incomplete cytoreduction is an obstructed ureter. This results from high-grade cancer progressing along the ureter, which is a retroperitoneal structure. There is a small likelihood of a complete resection with clear margins on the ureter and surrounding cancer. Ureteral resection or uretero-nephrectomy may be needed if all other sites of disease can be cleared (Figure 2.8).

In the resection of some colon and appendiceal cancers, the psoas muscle is the deep margin of resection. Minimal residual disease on the psoas muscle can progress as cancer infiltration of this muscle. With progression, deep infiltration along the fascicles of the psoas muscle may occur and is difficult to eradicate surgically (Figure 2.9). Complete resection of the psoas muscle may be required.

Concerning Radiologic Features Associated with of Peritoneal Metastases within the Pelvis

Surgical management of ovarian or rectal cancer may require generous removal of pelvic peritoneum. Also, resections of the pelvic sidewall lymph nodes are a standard part of primary ovarian cancer resections. Seeding of these deep pelvic dissections can result in a disease progression within the pelvic sidewall (Figure 2.10). This is difficult or usually impossible to resect even with a minimal margin. Also, encasement of common or external iliac vessels may preclude complete surgery.

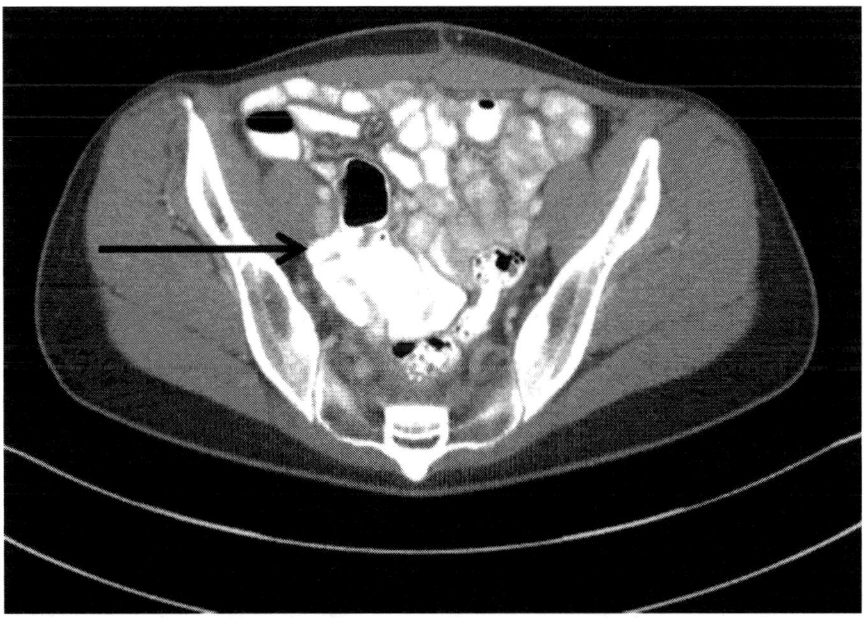

Figure 2.10. CT slice showing pelvic sidewall invasion. A patient with peritoneal mucinous carcinoma of appendiceal origin underwent pelvic lymphadenectomy and tumor reseeded on the right pelvic sidewall. At her first surgery she was thought to have ovarian cancer.

The rectouterine space in the female and rectovesical space in the male are sites of special concern for progression of peritoneal metastases. Stenosis of the mid-rectum can occur in the female patient with peritoneal metastases deep in the cul-de-sac. In the male, the peritoneal metastases can invade into the seminal vesicles (Figure 2.11A). The seminal vesicles are identified by the cross-sectional CT slice but nodules of tumor from the rectovesical peritoneum invade into and involve the seminal vesicles indicated by the absence of an intervening fat plane. On a CT section just above the seminal vesicles, tumor is lodged medially between the right and left seminal vesicles and is progressing as a layer of cancer within the peritoneum above the pararectal fossa (Figure 2.11B).

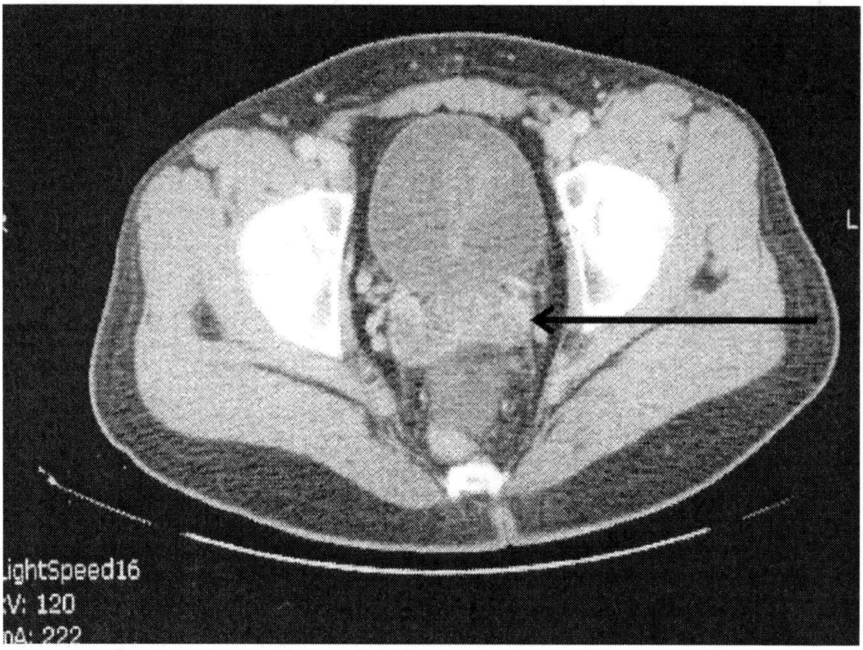

Figure 2.11A. CT slice showing peritoneal metastases between right and left seminal vesicle. A fat plane is absent.

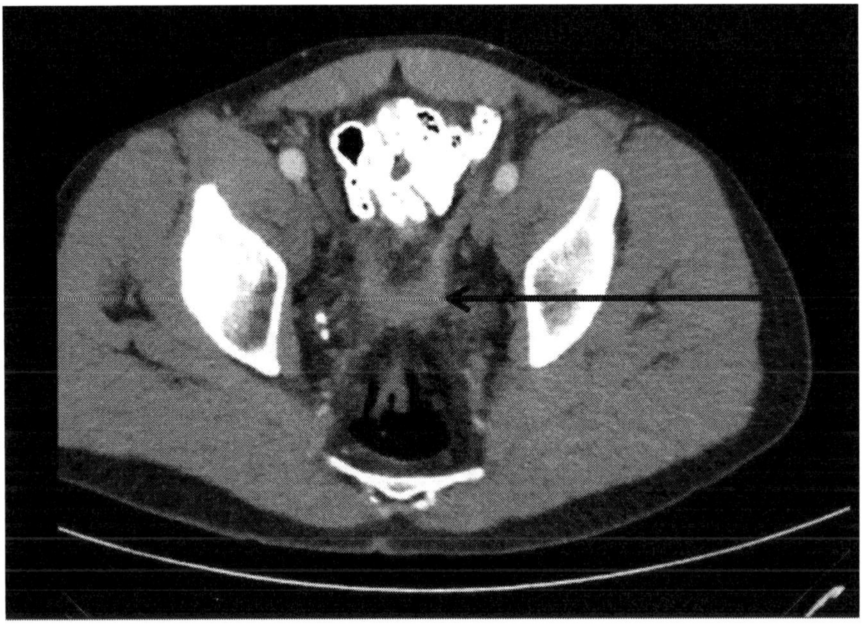

Figure 2.11B. CT slice a few millimeters above seminal vesicles with tumor layered out on peritoneum of pararectal fossa.

Recurrent invasive disease within the pelvis has profound implications for an optimal resection. Pelvic peritoneum, female internal genitalia, and rectosigmoid colon may need to be resected. Also, if the seminal vesicles are invaded, these must be resected which has implications for postoperative sexual function [14]. A peritoneal metastasis that involves the trigone of the bladder may preclude complete cytoreduction.

Concerning Radiologic Features Associated with Gastrohepatic or Hepatoduodenal Ligaments

The gastrohepatic ligament, subpyloric space, and hepatoduodenal ligaments are prominent sites for progression of peritoneal metastases. High-grade nodules with sclerotic capabilities may narrow or even occlude the common hepatic duct.

Cancer nodules on the posterior aspect of the hepatoduodenal ligament may involve the portal vein. It is important to identify tumor beneath the hepatic bridge that surrounds the round ligament of the liver. Failure to remove this tumor will result in obstruction of the left bile duct [15]. Large volume tumor in the gastrohepatic ligament may involve the left gastric artery (Figure 2.12). Partial or total gastrectomy may be required for complete cytoreduction.

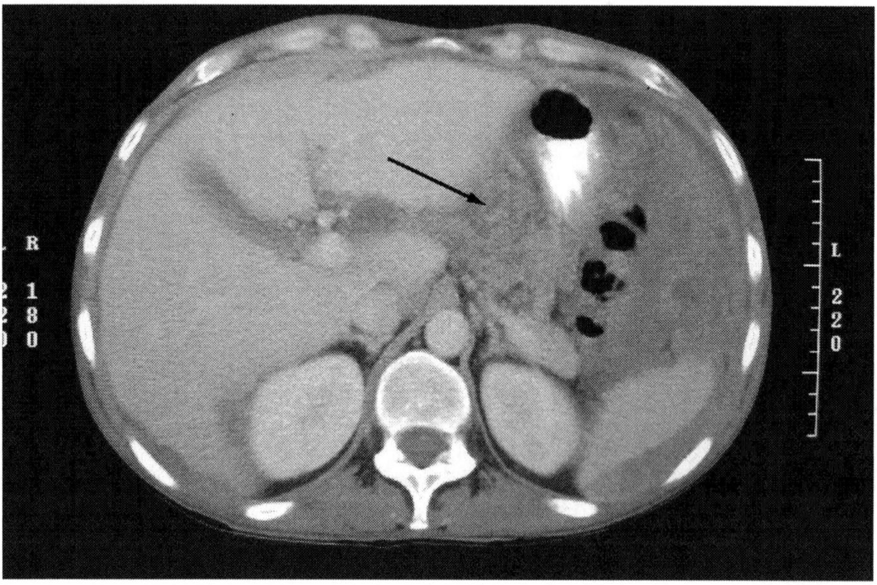

Figure 2.12. CT slice showing tumor ≥ 5 cm in diameter in gastrohepatic ligament.

Tumor cells entering through the Foramen of Winslow can lodge and progress within the lesser sac. Gastric outlet obstruction or partial obstruction may result from tumor accumulation on the fixed and immobile gastric antrum, pylorus, and first portion of the duodenum. Tumor accumulations anterior and posterior to the antrum of the stomach may result in gastric outlet obstruction (Figure 2.13).

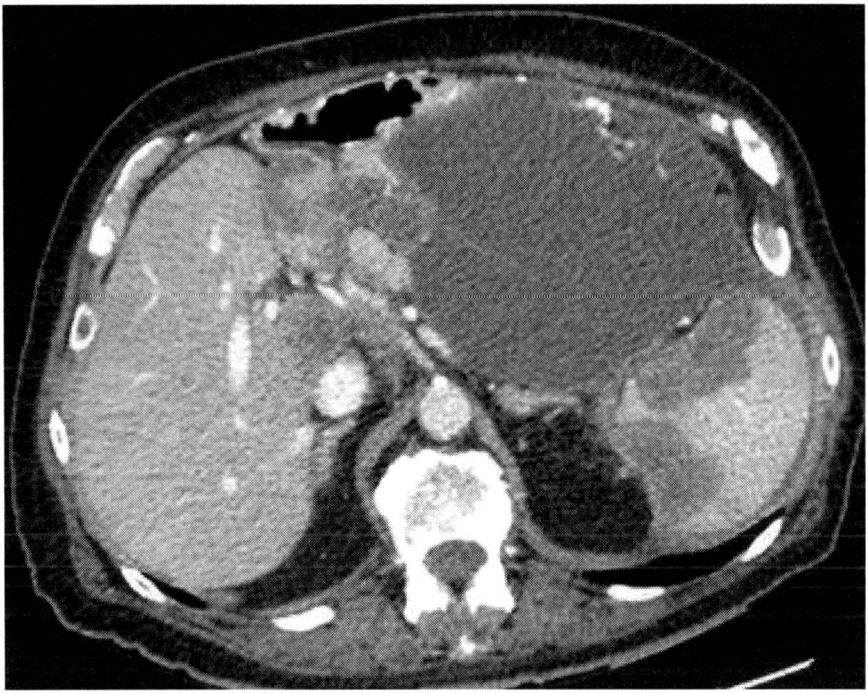

Figure 2.13. CT slice showing gastric outlet obstruction.

Concerning Radiologic Features Associated with Ascites

Hemorrhagic ascites in a cancer patient often indicates spontaneous necrosis of a high-grade tumor which may be indicative of diffuse peritoneal nodules throughout the abdomen. Most hemorrhagic ascites due to peritoneal metastases has attenuation values less than 30 Hounsfield Units (HU) with an appearance similar to serous ascites. Serous ascites (non-mucinous ascites) often arises from the surface of tumor nodules (Figure 2.14). The ascites accumulates because lymphatic stomata and lymphoid aggregates are obstructed by tumor and ascites that would normally be resorbed continues to accumulate. Mucinous ascites with compartmentalized small bowel is not a concerning radiologic feature. Also, extensive ascites with malignant peritoneal mesothelioma is expected. However, serous ascites or hemorrhagic ascites is often associated with diffuse and invasive nodules on bowel and mesenteric surfaces. Other causes of serous ascites such as cirrhosis should be considered and ruled out.

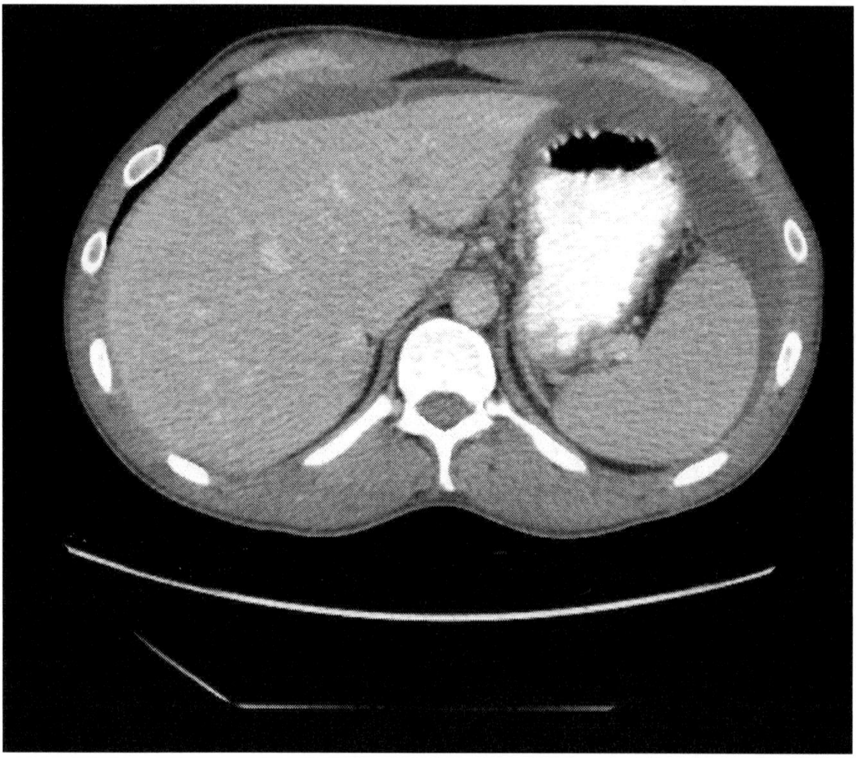

Figure 2.14. Extensive serous ascites in a gastrointestinal cancer patient.

Role for Laparoscopy

The major clinical implication of a concerning radiologic feature is to alert the multidisciplinary team to the possibility of an incomplete cytoreduction. Laparoscopy can be useful to confirm the high likelihood of an incomplete cytoreduction prior to planning a surgical intervention. Patients with a single concerning radiologic feature would become candidates for a laparoscopic exploration. If at the time of laparoscopy the extent of disease suggested complete cytoreduction, the management would proceed towards surgery. Alternatively, the combination of a single concerning radiologic feature with a concerning laparoscopic examination would suggest that cytoreductive surgery is not indicated.

Implications of One versus Two or More Concerning Radiologic Features

Jacquet et al. in 1995 reviewed CT parameters in 45 patients with known mucinous peritoneal metastases and described the CT findings. The 16 parameters they identified were statistically analyzed regarding their association with complete versus incomplete cytoreductive surgery. Both a single concerning CT finding and two CT findings were statistically analyzed regarding complete cytoreduction [16]. In a tree-structured analysis, patients who had obstruction of bowel segments by tumor and also tumor volume greater than 5 cm on proximal bowel surfaces had an incomplete cytoreduction 88% of the time. Those patients who had no obstruction of bowel segments and no tumor nodules greater than 0.5 cm on proximal small bowel had a 92% incidence of complete cytoreduction. In this study, the combination of two concerning radiologic features was strongly predictive of incomplete cytoreductive surgery. Yan et al. in 2004 studied 30 patients with malignant peritoneal mesothelioma [17]. They assessed the tumor extent by CT in 13 abdominopelvic regions and from 10 interpretative CT parameters. There was a 100% suboptimal cytoreduction if patients showed both tumor greater than 5 cm in the epigastric region and the interpretative assessment of small bowel and small bowel regions was class 3. In contrast, if the tumor size in the epigastric region was less than 5 cm and there were no class 3 interpretative findings in small bowel or small bowel mesentery, adequate cytoreduction was achieved in 94% of patients.

In a retrospective study of 15 patients Rivard et al. in 2014 critically evaluated preoperative CT and its implications for patient selection for treatment of peritoneal metastases. Although patients with a single concerning radiologic feature had the same percentage (87% versus 93%) of complete versus incomplete cytoreduction, those seven patients with two concerning radiologic features only had a single complete cytoreduction. This was significant with a p-value of 0.04 [18]. Finally, Yong et al. in 2016 evaluated unresectability of 172 consecutive patients who underwent CRS and HIPEC. They reported that abdominal distension from ascites, omental thickening, CT evidence of lymphadenopathy, and CT evidence for small bowel disease were all associated with a statistically significant incidence of incomplete cytoreduction. This group did not assess the implications of the presence of 1 versus 2 or more concerning radiologic features [19].

Conclusion

The concerning CT features we have identified are bowel obstruction at more than one site, mesentery drawn together by tumor, tumor infiltration between the leaves of the mesentery, tumor ≥5 cm in jejunal regions, CT peritoneal cancer index >20, mesenteric or para-aortic lymphadenopathy, hydroureter, psoas muscle invasion, porta hepatis infiltration, tumor >5 cm in gastrohepatic ligament or subpyloric space, gastric outlet obstruction, and/or hemorrhagic or serous ascites. These CT findings in a patient with peritoneal metastases are highly associated with incomplete cytoreductive surgery and suggest the need for diagnostic laparoscopy prior to a surgical intervention. Two concerning CT features has been shown to greatly increase the likelihood of an incomplete cytoreduction.

REFERENCES

[1] Glehen O, Gilly FN, Boutitie F, et al. Toward curative treatment of peritoneal carcinomatosis from nonovarian origin by cytoreductive surgery combined with reoperative intraperitoneal chemotherapy. *Cancer* 2010;116:5608-5618.

[2] O'Dwyer S, Verwaal VJ, Sugarbaker PH. Evolution of treatments for peritoneal metastases from colorectal cancer. *J Clin Oncol* 2015;33:2122.

[3] *Colon Cancer. Clinical Practice Guidelines in Oncology* (NCCN Guidelines). Version 2.2017 – 1/17/2018. Accessed at https://www.nccn.org/professionals/physician_gls/pdf/colon.pdf

[4] Elias D, Gilly F, Boutitie F, et al. Peritoneal colorectal carcinomatosis treated with surgery and perioperative intraperitoneal chemotherapy: Retrospective analysis of 523 patients from a multicentric French study. *J Clin Oncol* 2010;28:63-68.

[5] Sugarbaker PH, van der Speeten K. An overview of peritonectomy, visceral resection, and therapeutic laparoscopy for peritoneal surface malignancy. (In) Sugarbaker PH (Ed). *Cytoreductive Surgery & Perioperative Chemotherapy for Peritoneal Surface Malignancy. Textbook and Video Atlas.* 2nd Edition. Cine-Med Publishing: Woodbury, CT, 2017, pp. 17-46.

[6] Deraco M, Baratti D, Kusamura S, et al. Surgical technique of parietal and visceral peritonectomy for peritoneal surface malignancies. *J Surg Oncol* 2009;100:321-328.

[7] Sugarbaker PH. Peritoneum as the first line of defense in carcinomatosis. *J Surg Oncol* 2007;95(2):93-96.

[8] Sugarbaker PH, Averbach AM. Krukenberg syndrome as a natural manifestation of tumor cell entrapment. (In) Sugarbaker PH (ed). *Peritoneal Carcinomatosis: Principles of Management.* Kluwer: Boston, 1996, pp. 163-191.

[9] Sugarbaker PH, Sardi A, Brown G, Dromain C, Rousset P, Jelinek JS. Concerning CT features used to select patients for treatment of

peritoneal metastases, a pictoral essay. *Int J Hyperthermia* 33(5):497-504, 2017 DOI: 10.1080/02656736.2017.1317368.

[10] Jacquet P, Sugarbaker PH. Current methodologies for clinical assessment of patients with peritoneal carcinomatosis. *J Exp Clin Cancer Res* 1996;15(1):49-58.

[11] Esquivel J, Chua TC, Stojadinovic A, et al. Accuracy and clinical relevance of computed tomography scan interpretation of peritoneal cancer index in colorectal cancer peritoneal carcinomatosis: a multi-institutional study. *J Surg Oncol* 2010;102:565-570.

[12] Koh JL, Yan TD, Glenn D, Morris DL. Evaluation of pre-operative computed tomography in estimating peritoneal cancer index in colorectal peritoneal carcinomatosis. *Ann Surg Oncol* 2009;16:327-333.

[13] Archer AG, Sugarbaker PH, Jelinek JS. Radiology of peritoneal carcinomatosis. (In) Sugarbaker PH (ed). *Peritoneal Carcinomatosis: Principles of Management.* Kluwer: Boston, 1996, pp. 263-288.

[14] Sugarbaker PH. Peritoneal metastases invading the seminal vesicles: Radiologic appearance and outcome of treatment. *Eur J Surg Oncol* 2018;44(6):805-809.

[15] Sugarbaker PH. Pont Hepatique (Hepatic Bridge), an important anatomic structure in cytoreductive surgery. *J Surg Oncol* 2010;101:251-252.

[16] Jacquet P, Jelinek JS, Chang D, Koslowe P, Sugarbaker PH. Abdominal computed tomographic scan in the selection of patients with mucinous peritoneal carcinomatosis for cytoreductive surgery. *J Am Coll Surg* 1995;181:530-538.

[17] Yan TD, Haveric N, Carmignani P, Chang D, Sugarbaker PH. Abdominal computed tomography scans in the selection of patients with malignant peritoneal mesothelioma for comprehensive treatment with cytoreductive surgery and perioperative intraperitoneal chemotherapy. *Cancer* 2005;15:839-849.

[18] Rivard JD, Temple WJ, McConnell YJ, Sultan H, Mack LA. Preoperative computed tomography does not predict respectability in peritoneal carcinomatosis. *Am J Surg* 2014;207:760-765.

[19] Yong ZZ, Tan GH, Wong JF, Lim C, Soo KC, Teo MC. Unresectability during open surgical exploration in planned cytoreductive surgery and hyperthermic intraperitoneal chemotherapy. *Int J Hyperthermia* 2016;32(8):889-894.

In: Pictorial Essays … ISBN: 978-1-53618-014-5
Editors: PH Sugarbaker and RN Low ©2020 Nova Science Publishers, Inc.

Chapter 3

IDENTIFICATION OF PRIMARY COLORECTAL CANCER PATIENTS AT HIGH RISK FOR SURGICAL TREATMENT FAILURE AND EARLY DETECTION OF RECURRENT DISEASE

Gina Brown, MD, FRCR
Royal Marsden and Imperial College, London, UK

INTRODUCTION

Radiologic identification of the primary colon and upper rectal cancer patient, who is at high risk for local recurrence and peritoneal metastases, is the key to improved management. CT can identify patients at risk for surgical treatment failure that occurs because of local-regional and peritoneal disease. Patients with advanced primary cancer are likely to develop local and peritoneal recurrence [1, 2].

For example, in an advanced caecal tumor, even if the colorectal surgeon achieves an R0 resection, cancer progression in the right upper quadrant of the abdomen may occur with fatal consequences.

Identifying these high-risk cases at initial presentation, prior to the surgical intervention, is essential to optimize management decisions. The subsequent conversation between the patient, the surgeon and the multidisciplinary team prior to any surgical intervention will discuss possible treatments to reduce recurrence in these high-risk patients. The management of these patients should begin with a high-quality CT scan knowledgably interpreted to facilitate identifying the T3 and T4 cancers, which are at higher risk of local recurrence.

Identification of Primary Colorectal Cancer Patients at High Risk for Surgical Treatment Failure

Figure 3.1 shows a large partially obstructing right colon cancer. Although the CT scan is limited by lack of oral contrast material, one can appreciate the T stage of this tumor. The mass in the ascending colon is well visualized. In addition, the parietal and visceral peritoneum is abnormally thickened. Although peritoneal thickening on CT can be due to associated inflammation, in our experience in this clinical setting peritoneal inflammation and peritoneal tumor go hand in hand.

In the histologic section, the peri-inflammatory desmoplastic reaction is superimposed on a layer of cancer that is only micrometers thick. The preoperative oral contrast-enhanced CT does not over stage these cases with peritoneal thickening, because inflammation and peritoneal tumor are both typically present.

Identification of these high-risk patients predicts a poor prognosis with a 50% 3-year local relapse rate. Interestingly, even if the histopathology does not agree, our experience confirms that these patients with thick peritoneum at the primary colon cancer site are at high risk for local-regional surgical treatment failure.

The advanced sigmoid colon cancer (arrow) shown in the top part of Figure 3.2 is a mucinous tumor that also involves a portion of small bowel. In the lower part of Figure 2, one can see there is tumor growing along the veins (arrow). There is discontinuous vascular invasion in association with a mucinous colonic primary. This patient's tumor has a poor prognosis.

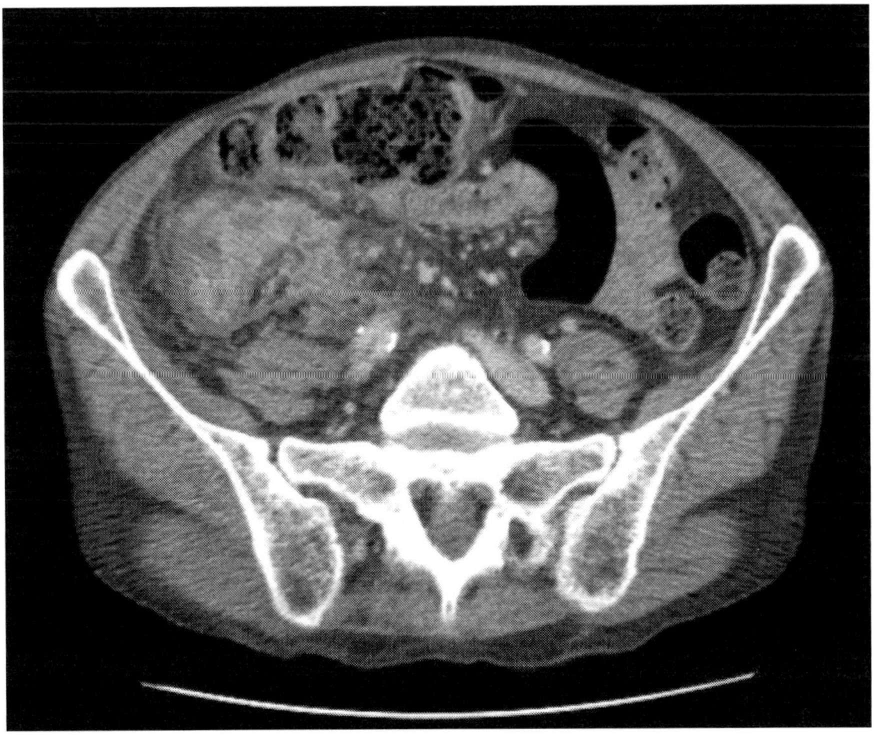

Figure 3.1. CT of a T4 primary ascending colon cancer. The peritoneum surrounding the tumor is irregular and thickened.

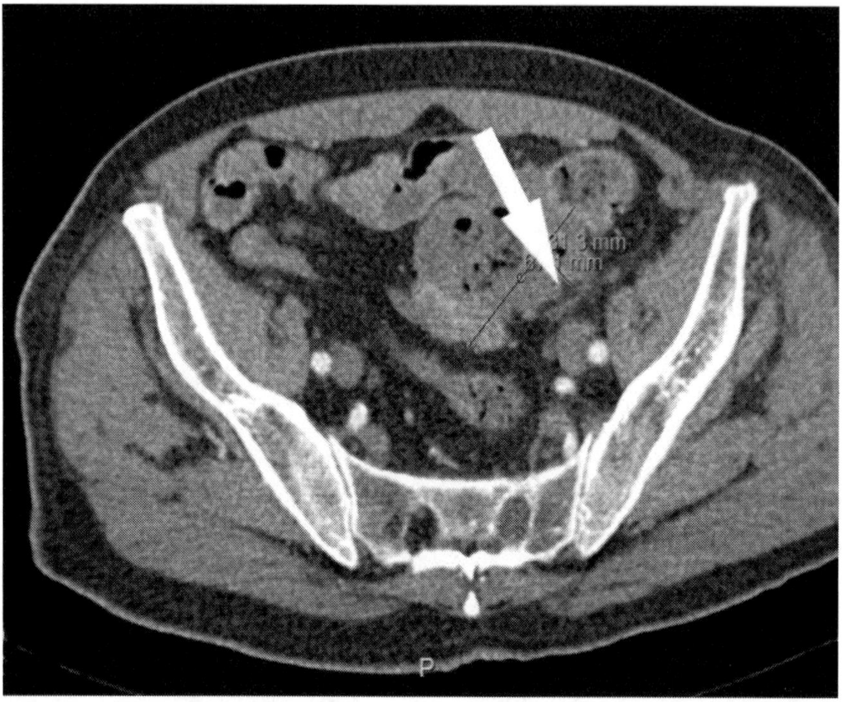

Figure 3.2 Top. An advanced mucinous sigmoid colon cancer involving a portion of small bowel.

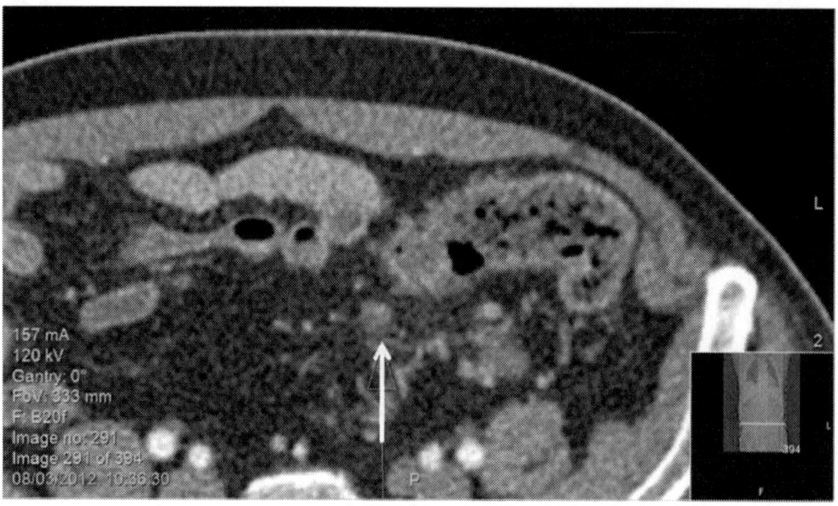

Figure 3.2 Bottom. The tumor is growing along the veins and nodular disease is outside the lymph nodes.

The decision to perform preoperative neoadjuvant chemotherapy should be discussed. The CT depicts vascular invasion and tumor encroachment upon the small bowel indicating a radiologic T4N1 tumor. The tumor could actually be considered T4N1c because of the nodular disease is outside of lymph nodes, which carries a worse prognosis. The histologic evaluation confirmed the radiologic findings in this patient. However, the pathology did not show venous invasion. This discordance of the radiologic findings and the pathology report occurs frequently. When there is discordance between the radiology and pathology reports, we can request the pathologist to re-review the specimens with attention to the radiologic findings, in this case the vascular invasion. A proforma radiologic report made available to the pathologist can assist him in the diligent search for the pathologic correlate of the disease identified on imaging,

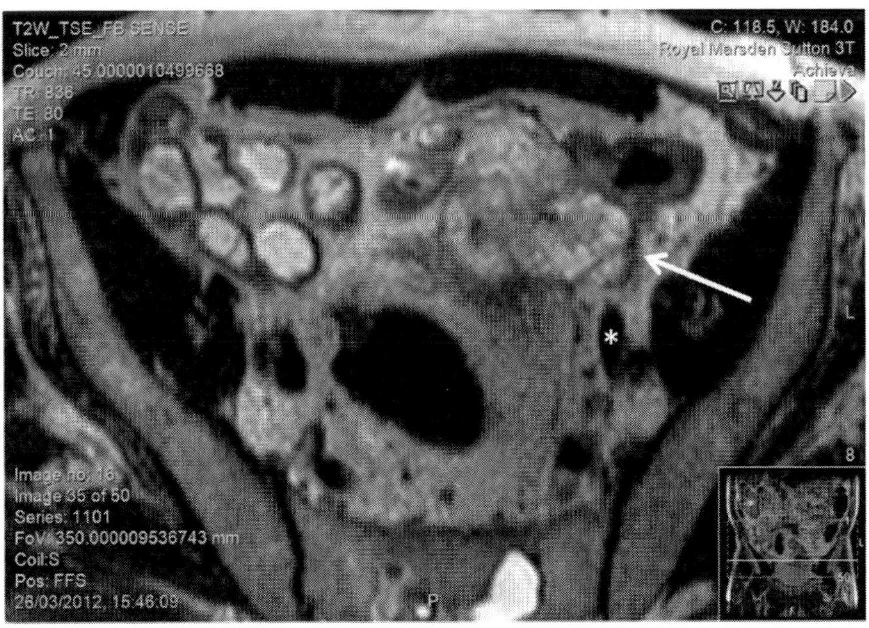

Figure 3.3. MRI of a sigmoid colon cancer with lateral extension to the pelvic sidewall. The asterisk is on left external iliac vein.

Figure 3.3 shows the equivalent MRI to the CT shown in Figure 3.2. The MRI depicts the mucinous tumor much more clearly than on the CT. On the MRI, we are seeing the extent of tumor and the primary cancer's proximity to the potential margins of resection.

We often consider the margins of a sigmoid colon cancer on the left pelvic sidewall as being relatively straightforward. Actually, in order to obtain a clear surgical margin and to avoid pelvic recurrence, this patient would need an extended dissection. The primary resection would need to include the parietal peritoneum and underlying fascia, which is not a routine resection for sigmoid cancer.

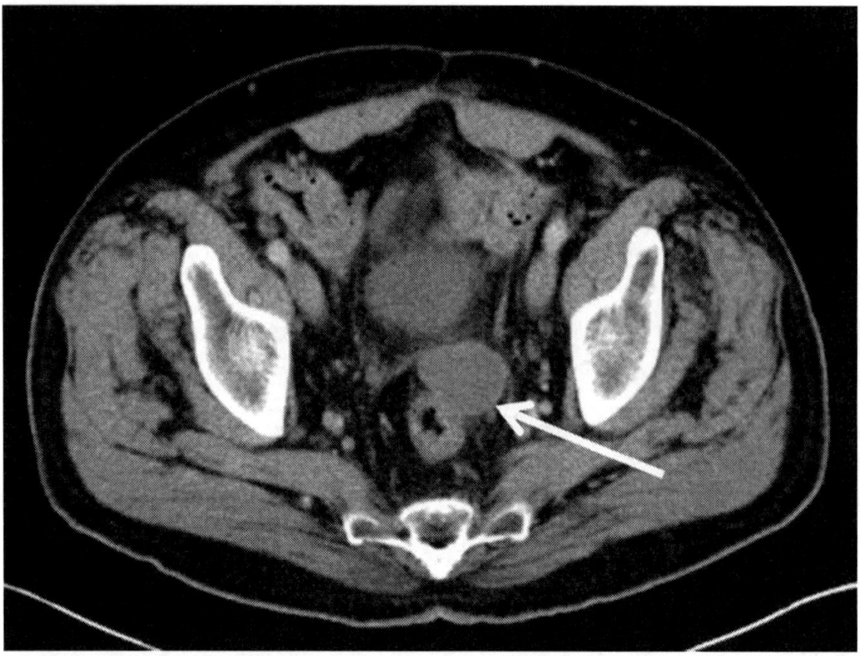

Figure 3.4. A primary mid-rectal cancer radiologically staged as T4N1c.

A preoperative discussion of extent of the primary cancer resection must occur in order to avoid suboptimal resection and tumor recurrence.

Preventing pelvic recurrence is an important goal of preoperative imaging and the subsequent discussion between surgeon, radiologist, and the multidisciplinary team. Many peritoneal recurrences can be prevented with a more precise surgical strategy using peritonectomy and an extended resection. These recurrences are a result of inadequate margins of resection and tumor spillage [3].

Figure 3.4 shows an upper rectal cancer with an extensive primary tumor but no evidence of peritoneal spread. The radiologist's report must describe the morphology of the tumor, its border and its location.

The advancing edge of the tumor should be described as being mesenteric or peritoneal. The tumor's relationship to the bowel wall should be described as intramural or transmural if it extends through the intestinal wall. It is known that transmural tumor extension more than 5mm portends a poor patient outcome.

Radiologic Identification of Poor Prognosis Sigmoid Colon Cancers

Sigmoid colon cancers are a problematic group of tumors. Sigmoid colon cancer makes up about a third of the total number of colon cancers so tackling sigmoid cancers as aggressively as we have tackled rectal cancers is worthwhile.

However, even anatomic localization is imprecise with important clinical consequences. A radiologist may report a rectal cancer as rectosigmoid leading the oncologist to treat it as a sigmoid colon cancer rather than a rectal cancer. The surgeon may classify the same tumor as a high rectal tumor and perform a partial TME. Since sigmoid colon cancer falls in between rectal and colon categories, the multidisciplinary team may not be able to determine the precise management plan.

Currently, in the United Kingdom we see a much higher local recurrence rate with sigmoid colon cancers as compared to rectal cancers, yet they are only separated by a couple of centimeters. It makes logical sense to regard sigmoid colon cancers in the same way as we have rectal cancers. That means preoperative staging and preoperative therapy because these sigmoid tumors are amenable to preoperative chemoradiotherapy or chemotherapy alone. They are also amenable to TME-type surgical resections. For example, the primary tumors are amenable to multi-visceral resections if they are staged and the patient and surgeon are prepared for an extended resection. A preoperative MRI may show the primary cancer invading the bladder or the pelvic sidewall.

For the surgeon to consider all sigmoid cancers as an easy and curative resection is incorrect and dangerous, because the outcome data confirms that these are not simple resections. Many of the potential disastrous outcomes are avoidable. A primary mid-sigmoid cancer may involve the non-peritonealized fascial margin. If the circumferential radial margin is involved, there is no surgeon who is going to be able to perform a primary resection on this tumor and obtain clear margins. Surgery alone is not the answer. If one can identify these patients preoperatively, additional therapy such as a preoperative targeted boost of radiotherapy at the positive margin could be considered. We must radiologically stage these sigmoid tumors preoperatively to identify the patients at high risk for local-regional recurrent disease. I am convinced that preoperative treatment would result in substantial improvements in outcome in approximately a third of patients with sigmoid colon cancer.

MRI in Sigmoid Colon Cancer Patients

We performed an evaluation of a series of patients that inadvertently had MRIs because their tumors were staged by their colonoscopist as being in the rectum when in fact they were in the sigmoid colon. It turns out that this mistake was fortunate for those patients. When they were scanned, we identified that some of these patient's tumors had radiologically positive margins. For these sigmoid colon cancer patients, we recommend primary chemoradiotherapy. We also identified patients inadvertently scanned who had the same poor prognostic features, and underwent primary surgery thinking there was no indication to give those sigmoid tumors preoperative therapy.

In total, we found 57 patients with preoperative MRI who underwent primary surgery of which 18 had a positive margin. In 37 patients the preoperative MR predicted a favorable prognosis. In 31 of the 37 patients the histopathologic findings concurred. In 6 tumors there was some disagreement with the primary histology. The tumors that we thought were poor prognosis on MRI showed concordance with the histopathology in about 50% of cases.

When we looked at the survival outcomes for these patients, the good MRI prognosis group had an excellent survival outcome. The poor MRI prognosis group which received radiotherapy for margin positive disease has had the same survival as the good prognosis group. The poor MRI prognosis group that didn't receive any radiotherapy has had a substantially significantly worse survival. These results suggest that there is benefit from treating the poor prognosis sigmoid colon cancer patients identified on MRI by more aggressive preoperative treatments. This is the basis for the FOXTROT trial looking at whether poor prognosis patients benefitted from an aggressive preoperative treatment strategy [3]. If these patients radiologically determined to have high risk sigmoid colon cancers receive preoperative chemoradiotherapy, perhaps they will do better in the future.

EARLY DETECTION OF RECURRENT DISEASE

The second part of this book chapter concerns the radiologic findings with recurrent colorectal cancer. Recurrence is often in the rectovesical pouch, exactly where one might expect it to be from a T4 tumor. The recurrence shown in Figure 3.5 was not identified on the first CT but rather on a second CT which showed interval enlargement. With mucinous tumors, early mucinous recurrence can appear as an accumulation of fluid within the peritoneal space. Reformatted CT images in the coronal and sagittal projections are essential to determine the location of the fluid collections as extra intestinal, leading to the correct diagnosis of recurrent mucinous tumor.

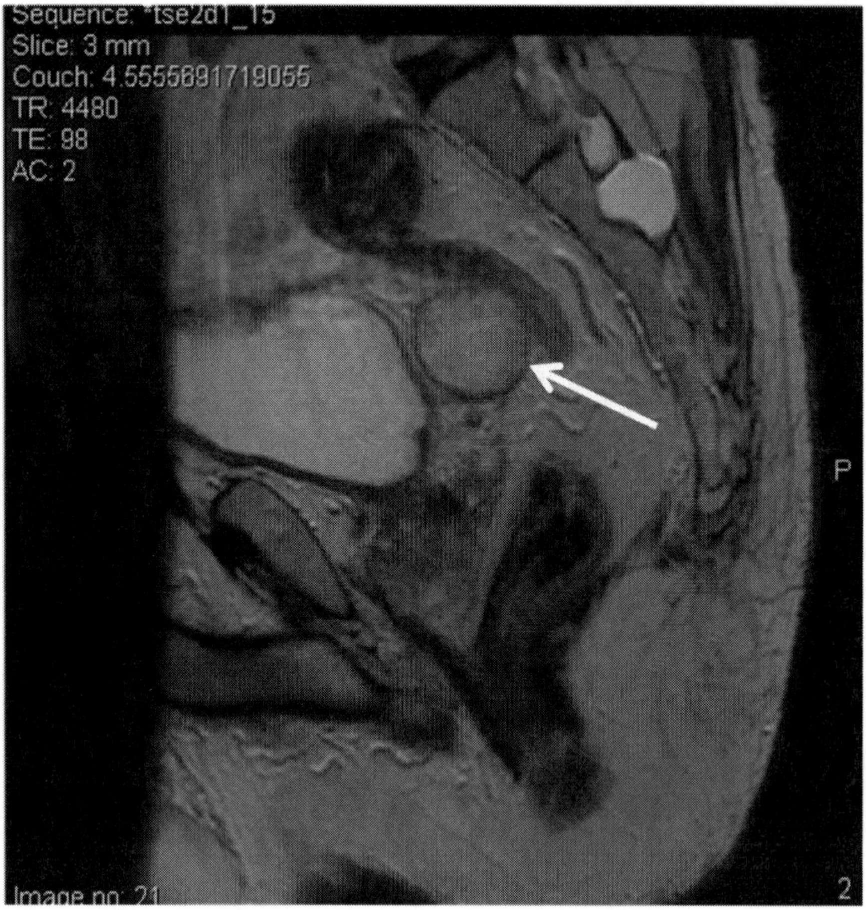

Figure 3.5. A T4 colon cancer that has recurred within the rectovesical pouch. Sagittal MRI slice show a well encapsulated deposit of partly necrotic moderately differentiated mucinous adenocarcinoma that lies between the bladder and the rectum. The tumor pushes up to the external border of the rectal muscularis propria. There is no invasion of the bladder wall or the ureter. A Tarlov cyst is present at S2, S3 (white arrow).

Figures 3.5 and 3.6 show the same pelvic mass on MRI that was poorly imaged by CT. The recurrent mass on MRI is clearly depicted and has a mucinous appearance. These are often referred to as "drop metastases" since they have occurred through peritoneal seeding and gravity distribution into the rectovesical pouch. These tumors are typically isolated with a more favorable prognosis. In this case recurrent mucinous tumor measures 6 cm by the time it was detected radiologically. However, it is localized to a single central compartment leading to a straightforward surgical resection. Radiologic diagnosis of recurrent (persistent and progressive disease) colorectal cancer can be a challenge, particularly in the pelvis. If there is doubt on CT regarding a pelvic recurrence, it is important to perform a pelvic MRI. A negative pelvic CT may be falsely reassuring but does not preclude tumor recurrence. Pelvic MRI should be performed in these patients for more optimal imaging and better patient management.

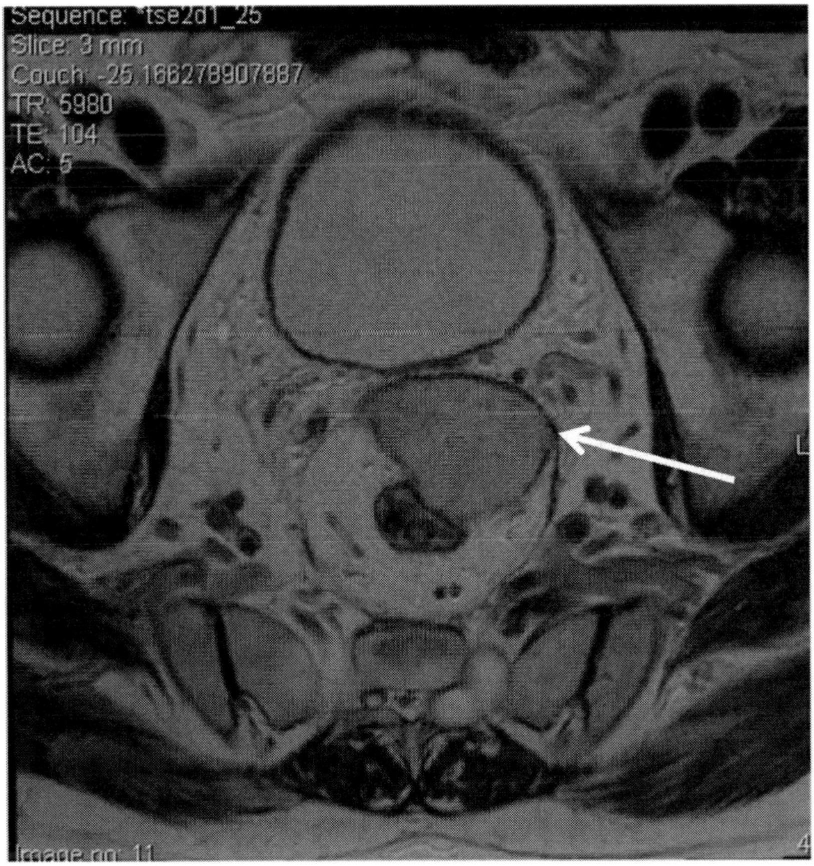

Figure 3.6. Transvers MRI slice shows no venous invasion. No tumor is seen in the small lymph nodes examined. Tumor is 1.8 mm from the left lateral resection margin but all other margins are clear of tumor (same patient as Figure 3.5).

Abnormal Pelvic Compartments by CT

Even with normal pelvic anatomy on CT scan, a collection of pelvic fluid should alert the radiologist to the possibility of tumor nodules lining the peritoneal compartment. It is necessary to determine the regional anatomy of the abdominal pelvic compartments. Regional anatomy by CT is important in terms of dividing the abdomen and pelvis into sections. These anatomic compartments are important to help determine the surgical procedures required to resect recurrent disease, whether it is the omental compartment, the central compartment in the rectum, i.e., the mesorectum, or whether it is the pelvirectal space. The contents of these compartments need to be considered and when tumor extends into more than one compartment, the surgery becomes more complex and requires a heightened assessment of surgical morbidity and mortality. Disease that is only involving the pouch of Douglas or the rectovesical space may be limited no matter what its size and may be amenable to resection. Tumor that has extended into the next compartment, which is the pelvirectal space, will need additional dissection. Further laterally, the pelvic compartment is bounded by the pelvic sidewall fascia. Disease at this site would require additional dissection. The procedures would be more difficult because they involve a vascular compartment including the internal and external iliac vessels and obturator nerve. Further laterally still, you then are dealing with the bony compartment which, for most surgeons, is a "no go" zone. I am convinced that compartmental anatomy should be described as we try to radiologically stage the extent and anatomic location of recurrent colon cancer. For example, if tumor is in the mesenteric compartment it may not be operable because of vascular encasement that limits the possibility of resection without devascularizing the abdominal contents. Radiologic description of extent and anatomic location by compartments is an essential first step.

Benefits of Comparison to Prior Studies

For the radiologic diagnosis of colorectal cancer recurrence, subtle changes in areas of peritoneal disease must be expected. With the 1 mm, 2½ mm, and 5 mm slices one can start to see disease on peritoneal surfaces.

By comparing the current examination to previous scans, even ones obtained one or two years previously, it becomes easier to appreciate subtle changes that may indicate recurrent tumor.

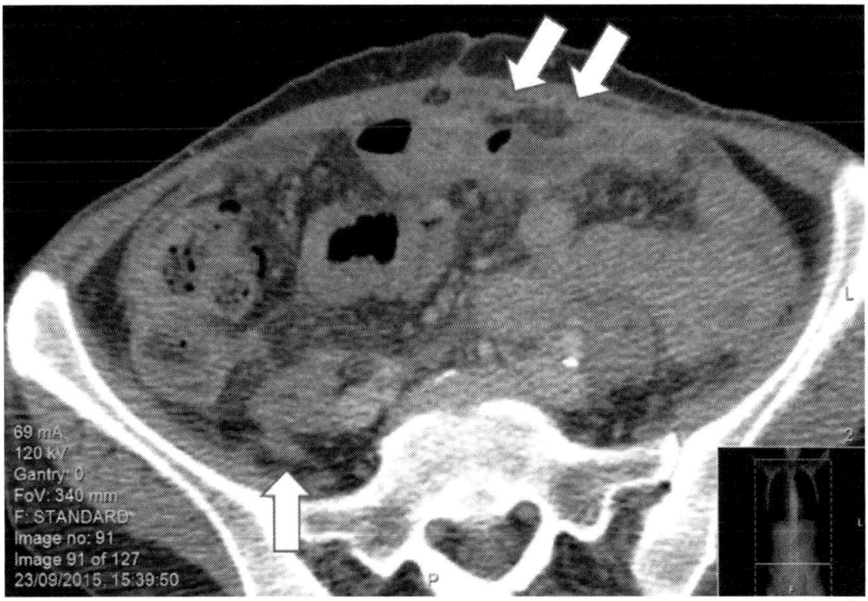

Figure 3.7. Subtle radiologic changes can be identified by comparison to prior studies. A baseline study is crucial for early radiologic identification of recurrent disease.

Particularly with a patient with a rising CEA or another tumor marker, the radiologist cannot be content with just looking at the most recent scan. Evaluation of serial radiologic studies is mandatory. Sometimes performing these comparisons does require extra effort to obtain copies of all prior CT examinations. Clinical information indicating rising tumor markers, or clinical concern about recurrence due to very marginal resection placing an anatomic site at “high risk” should alert the radiologist. The added time and effort to obtain a prior study will pay dividends if the radiologist can then detect subtle changes that indicate insidiously growing tumors. Actually, that insidious growth may be a good prognostic factor and may indicate the possibility of a surgical cure. Subtle 2 or 3 mm changes may become significant.

In Figure 3.7, one might not detect anything very obvious. However, if you compare this CT scan to a baseline CT, the rectus muscle has changed. There is a subtle tumor deposit sitting just under the rectus abdominis muscle and in the right paracolic space.

In this case the rising serum CEA and the positive PET scan alerted the radiologist to the fact that the patient had recurrence of tumor. Comparison of the baseline and the current CT are essential to detect these subtle changes.

Prognostic Implications for Reoperative Surgery of a Radiologic Assessment by Compartments

I am convinced that the “synoptic report” required for pelvic reporting can be adapted to the other abdominal compartments. The success of this approach of synoptic reporting is based upon the radiologist’s assessment of the distorted anatomy within each of the abdominal and pelvic compartments. One cannot overlook findings because one must make a decision about what is going on in the individual compartments. Interpretation starts with a knowledge of the etiology of the recurrent tumor.

1. Compartments Involved: In Figure 3.8 we proposed that the recurrent disease was of peritoneal origin because it ascended from the rectouterine pouch (pouch of Douglas) in a female patient.

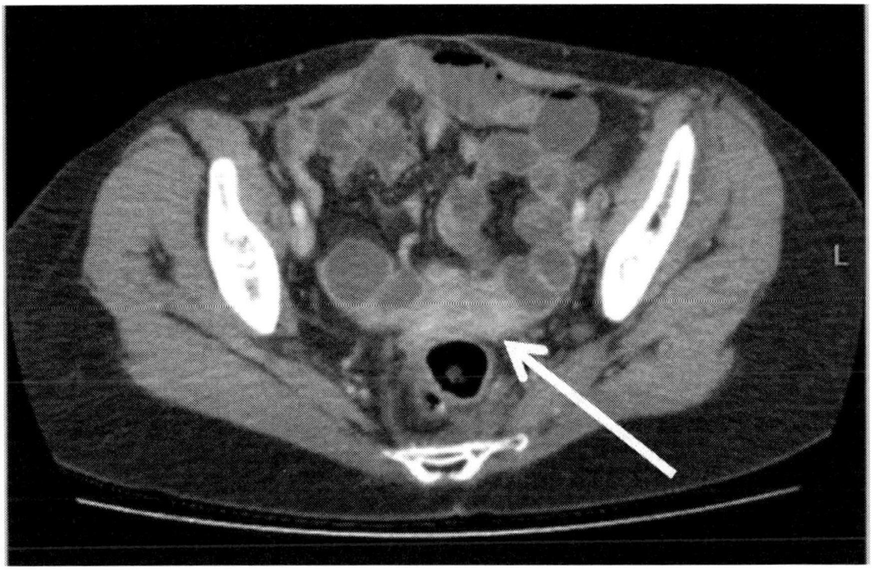

Figure 3.8. Radiologic identification of a recurrence within the rectouterine space in a female.

2. Unifocal vs Multifocal: We describe whether the tumor is unifocal or multifocal. We thought in this case that the tumor was multifocal.
3. Measurements: We provide measurements of the lesions because that is helpful in assessing response to therapy.
4. Evaluation of Other Compartments: We also evaluate each of the other compartments. The first compartment is above the peritoneal reflection but within the pelvis but it can extend into the abdomen. In this patient, the peritoneal infiltration involves small bowel loops and the base of the caecum.
5. Contiguous Anatomy: We then describe which anatomic structures the tumor abuts. In this case we thought it was pressing on the uterus and there was a possible left adnexal mass. Posteriorly, there was no involvement because none of the bony landmarks were involved by tumor. Laterally, there was no extension into the lateral sidewall compartments and there was no pelvic sidewall adenopathy.

6. Involvement of the Infralevator Compartment: The critical infralevator compartment will determine whether or not the patient would have an exenterative procedure that involves the removal of the sphincter complex.
7. Urogenital and Perineal Triangles: Finally, we examine the urogenital and perineal triangles.
8. Distant Peritoneal Metastases: We review the abdominal CT to look for peritoneal nodules elsewhere within the peritoneal cavity.

Radiologically, in this patient, 3 compartments were involved. The rectouterine pouch, bowel immediately adjacent to the pelvis, and the uterus and left adnexa. Consequently, the prognosis is guarded for complete resection with reoperation. The radiology report will indicate where the margins of complete resection are going to be.

The report would read as follows, “Based on the anatomy and the extent of disease that we can see, the patient would need an en-bloc removal of the pouch of Douglas mass with the adjacent uterus, vagina, and ovaries because we are not certain those are clear of disease. A segment of small bowel resected en-bloc may be required. There would not be a requirement to remove the bladder or to dissect the pelvic sidewall or to remove the sacrum. A central compartment resection would be required to achieve clear margins”.

At the time of surgery our prediction using this compartment assessment was correct in that the areas that we said were involved by tumor were invaded by recurrent cancer. The patient underwent an R0 resection and fortunately has not relapsed since. This case illustrates that the normal imaging report is insufficient. We need to focus more on the anatomy, compartments involved and the surgical planes. Our report provides the surgeon with an overview of what will be required to be resected in order to achieve an R0 resection.

REFERENCES

[1] Balyasnikova, S., Brown, G. Imaging advances in colorectal cancer. *Curr. Colorectal Cancer Rep.,* 2016; 12:162 - 169.

[2] Dighe, S., Blake, H., Koh, M.-D., Swift, I., Arnaout, A., Temple, L., Barbachano, Y., Brown, G. Accuracy of multidetector computed tomography in identifying poor prognostic factors in colonic cancer. *Br. J. Surg.,* 2010; 97:1407 - 1415.

[3] Foxtrot Collaborative Group. Feasibility of preoperative chemotherapy for locally advanced, operable colon cancer: the pilot phase of a randomised controlled trial. *Lancet Oncol.,* 2012; 13(11): 1152 - 1160.

In: Pictorial Essays ... ISBN: 978-1-53618-014-5
Editors: PH Sugarbaker and RN Low ©2020 Nova Science Publishers, Inc.

Chapter 4

DESCRIPTION OF PERITONEAL METASTASES BY MRI

Pascal Rousset, MD, PhD
Department of Radiology, Lyon Sud University Hospital, Lyon, France

INTRODUCTION

The role of MRI in peritoneal malignancy has significantly improved due to technical improvements as well as new MRI protocols [1, 2]. MRI is clearly an effective and well-established technique routinely used in many centers. MRI may help the radiologist respond to the diagnostic and therapeutic challenges which are to provide a timely diagnosis in the initial workup and to report any detection of tumor recurrence for the patient in surveillance. In addition, MRI can provide a preoperative assessment of the extent of the peritoneal metastases to assist in patient selection for potentially curative treatment.

PERITONEAL MRI READING

For optimal application of MRI the radiologist needs to combine the information from morphological sequences, including T2-weighted and gadolinium-enhanced images, with the functional diffusion-weighted images [3]. The final report is a synthesis of all of the MRI information, which will optimally depict and characterize all peritoneal lesions.

Peritoneal Metastases MRI Using T2-Weighted Images

The reading can start with the T2-weighted sequences, which are very useful because it gives anatomic details that can display all the structures and that helps us to precisely localize the different lesions. Figure 4.1 left shows non-mucinous lesions with an intermediate signal in the T2-weighted sequence in the pouch of Douglas. The lesions are not so easy to depict on CT (Figure 4.1 middle). Figure 4.1 right is an intraoperative photograph documenting three peritoneal metastases at the precise anatomic location indicated by MRI and CT.

In contrast, T2-weighted images are very useful and efficient to depict mucinous lesions because of their fluid content within a cystic nodule. In Figure 4.2 one can see the small lesion from a mucinous colorectal cancer, less than 5 mm, in contact with the diaphragm. It was retrospectively present on CT but more difficult to see.

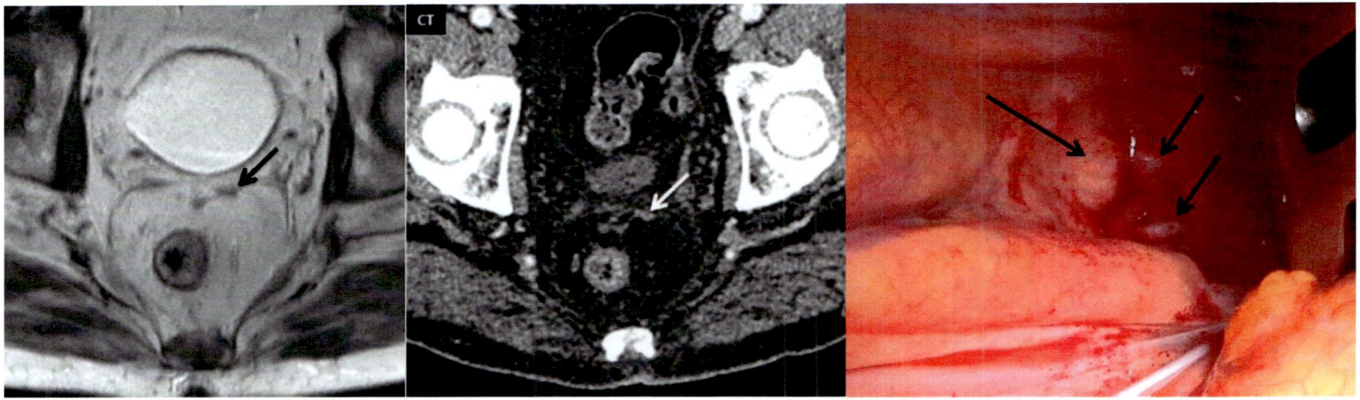

Figure 4.1. Shows three peritoneal nodules in the pouch of Douglas on MRI and CT, confirmed at surgery (black arrows).

Peritoneal Metastases Imaged by Gadolinium-Enhanced MRI Sequences

Post-contrast morphological sequences of gadolinium-enhanced MRI display well thickening of parietal peritoneum [4]. Figure 4.3 shows delayed fat suppressed gadolinium-enhanced MRI sequences.

They are very useful in reading because they can demonstrate nodules and fat stranding, but most of all, peritoneal thickening. These post-contrast sequences can clearly depict the parietal peritoneum as seen in Figure 4.3 in the posterior part of the pelvis. Figure 4.4 shows axial CT and a gadolinium-enhanced MRI image from a patient with malignant peritoneal mesothelioma. MRI displays not only the malignant involvement but it also helps to differentiate it from the normal diaphragm because of the high contrast resolution of MRI, which is very difficult on CT.

The coronal plane is very useful to depict lesions in the mesentery, the paracolic gutter, as well as on the undersurface of the hemidiaphragm. In Figure 4.5, there was only a 1 week interval between the CT and MRI examinations. The thick enhancement of the right diaphragm is clearly best seen on MRI when compared to the CT.

Post-contrast morphological sequences of gadolinium-enhanced MRI also displays well thickening of visceral peritoneum. The patient shown in Figure 4.6 had unresectable ovarian cancer due to diffuse infiltration of the visceral peritoneum of the liver, spleen, and anterior part of the stomach, that was well displayed on MRI as compared to CT.

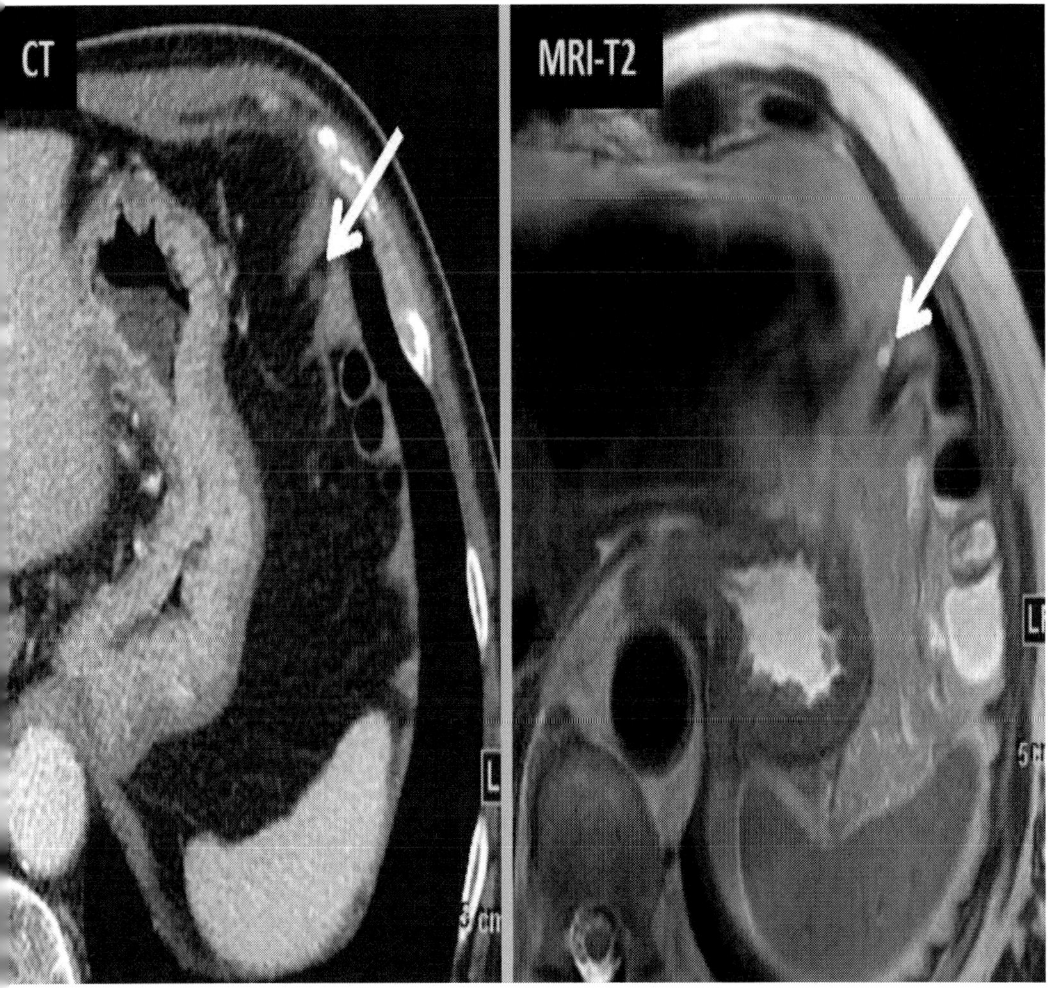

Figure 4.2. Shows a small lesion in contact with the left hemidiaphragm (arrows) better seen on T2-weighted sequence than retrospectively on CT.

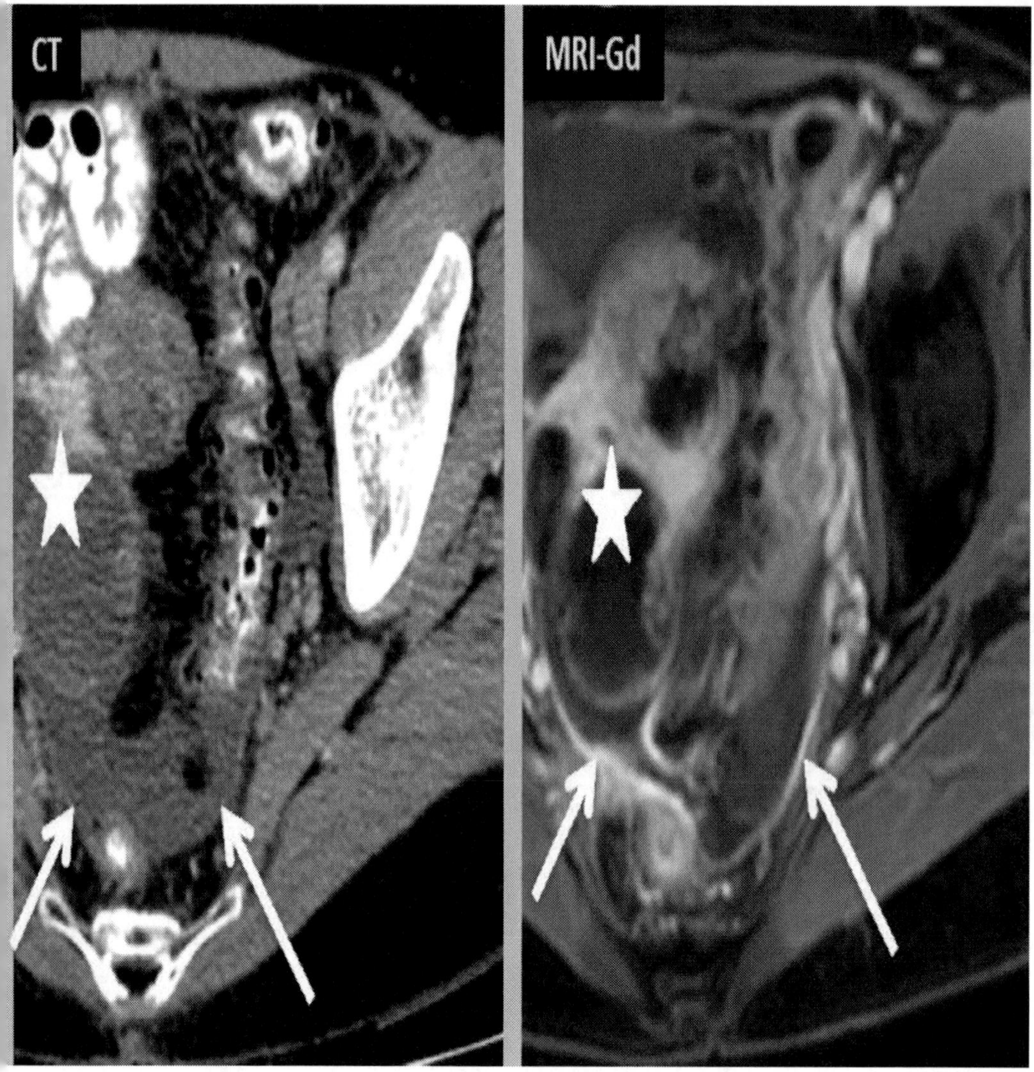

Figure 4.3. CT and delayed fat-suppressed gadolinium-enhanced MRI sequences. Malignant thickenings more than 3 mm thick appear more or less irregular (arrows) well displayed on MRI and not clearly seen on CT in this patient with an ovarian cancer (stars).

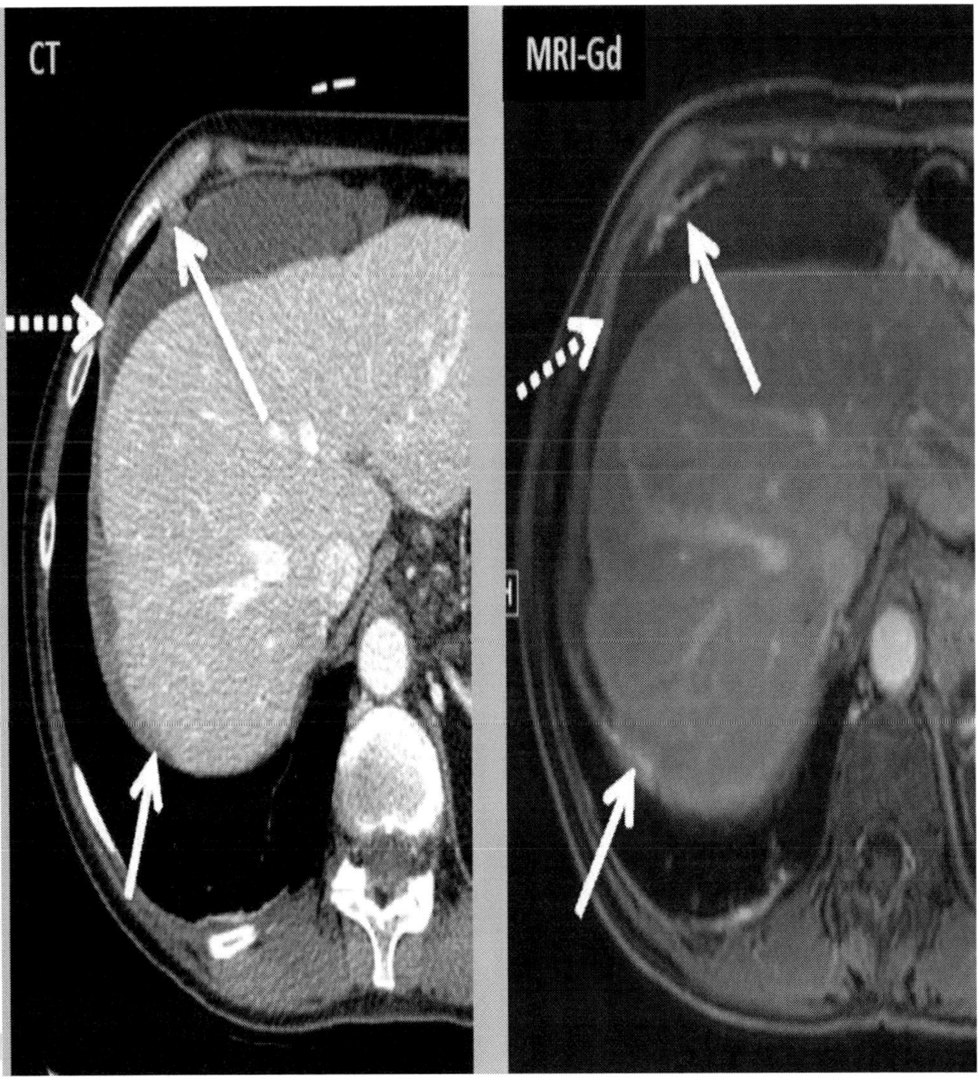

Figure 4.4. In this patient with malignant peritoneal mesothelioma, the lesions are clearly depicted on MRI (arrows) and are well differentiated from the normal diaphragm (dashed arrows). This is much less obvious on CT.

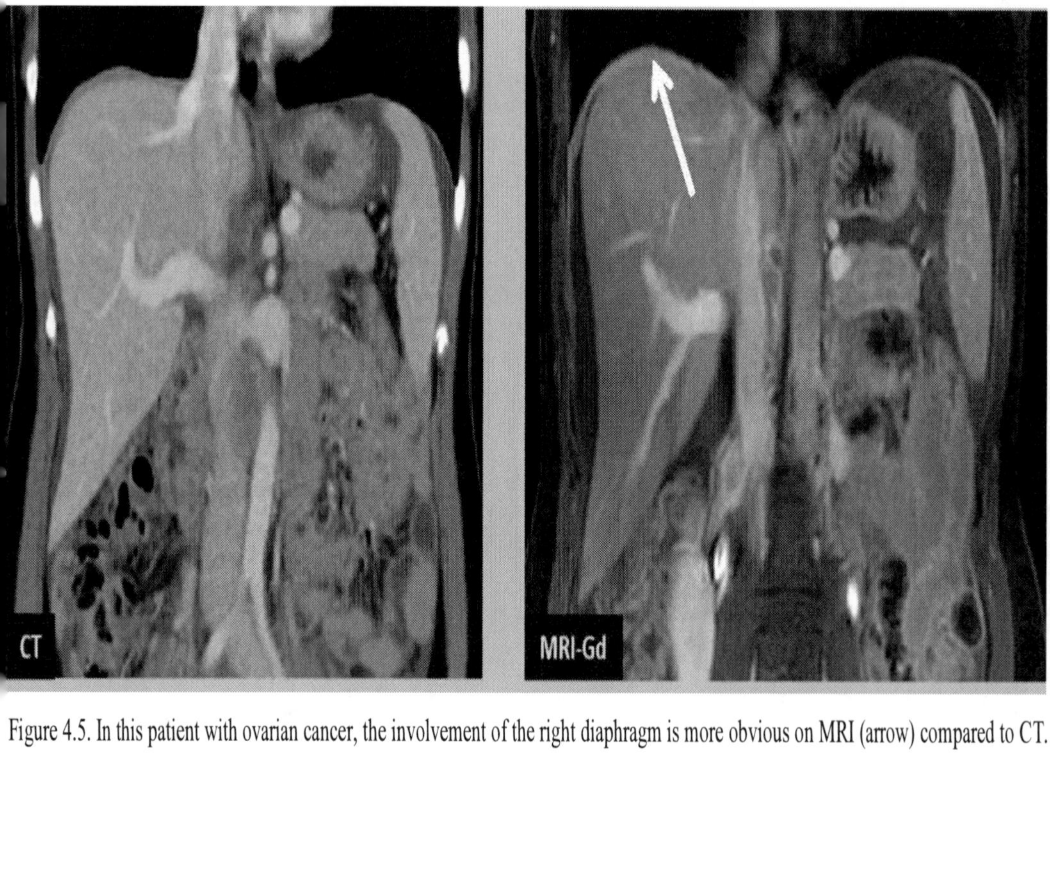

Figure 4.5. In this patient with ovarian cancer, the involvement of the right diaphragm is more obvious on MRI (arrow) compared to CT.

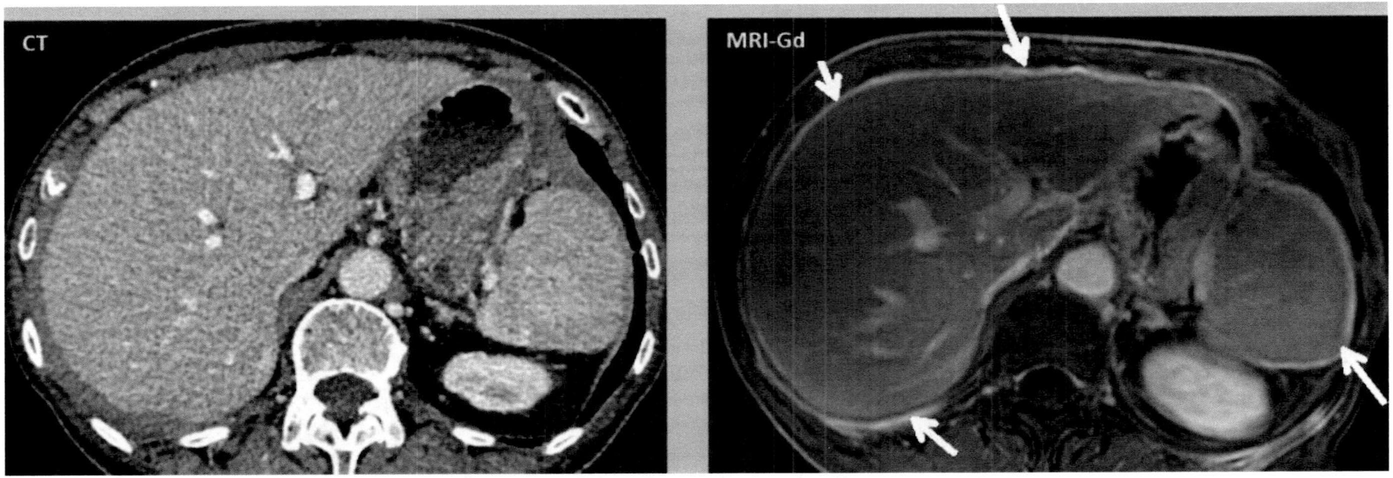

Figure 4.6. In this patient with ovarian cancer, gadolinium-enhanced MRI sequences are very efficient to show visceral peritoneum involvement. CT does not show that this woman had unresectable diffuse thickening of the visceral peritoneal surfaces of the whole upper abdomen. On MRI, there is diffuse and thick peritoneal involvement of the whole upper abdomen including perihepatic involvement (arrows).

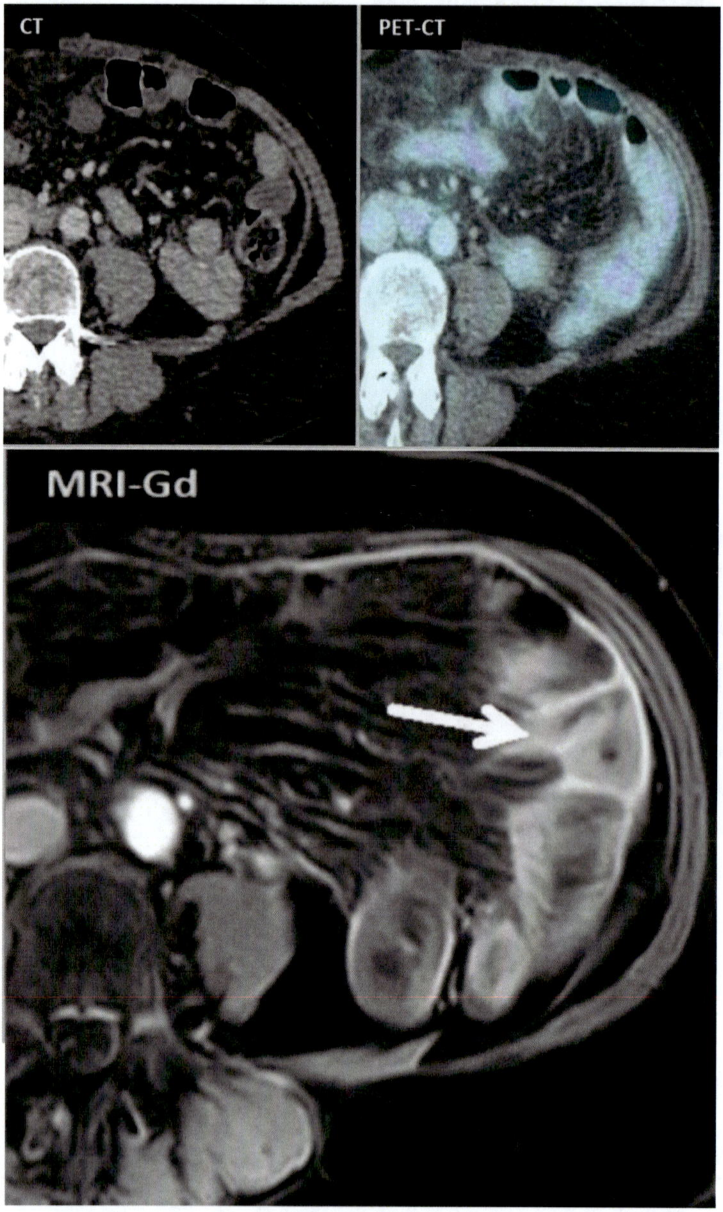

Figure 4.7A. Left. In this patient with malignant peritoneal mesothelioma, CT, PET-CT and MRI were performed within the 3 days before surgery and only MRI provided information on the proximal jejunum involvement with an irregular thickening of the small bowel serosa and its mesenteric border (arrow).

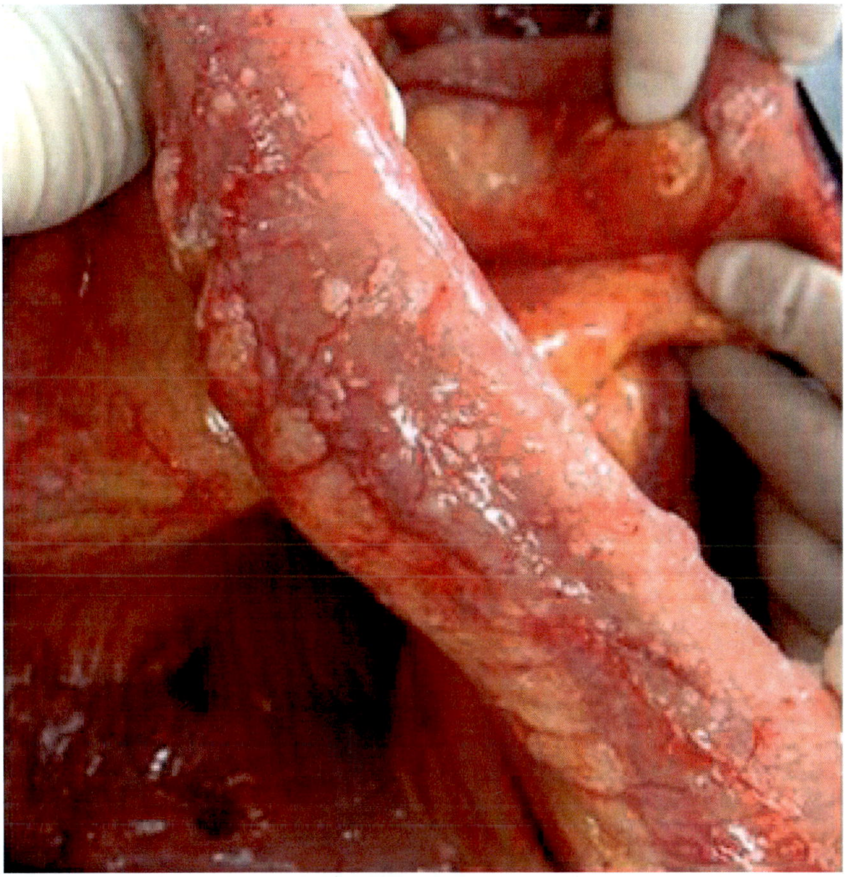

Figure 4.7B. Right. An intraoperative photograph.

Involvement of the small bowel and its mesentery is critical for patient selection and MRI is very useful for this indication. The patient studied in Figure 4.7A had all three radiologic techniques (CT, PET-CT and MRI) performed three days before surgery. MRI depicted the enhancement of the jejunum with a thick, more or less irregular bowel serosa, and mesenteric border enhancement. This layering of tumor was present at surgery (Figure 4.7B). Neither CT nor PET-CT showed these changes.

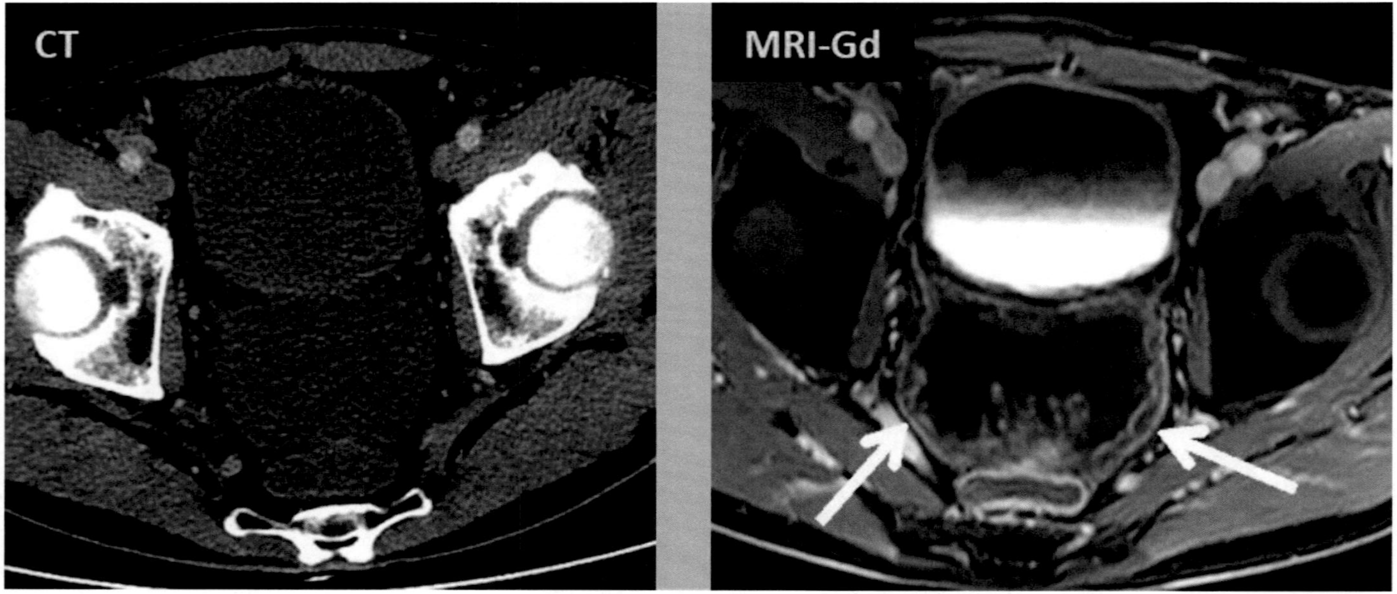

Figure 4.8. In this patient with pseudomyxoma peritonei, CT cannot differentiate mucinous ascites from mucinous tissue. MRI with gadolinium injection shows a thick and diffuse peritoneal tissue enhancement lining the pelvis (arrows).

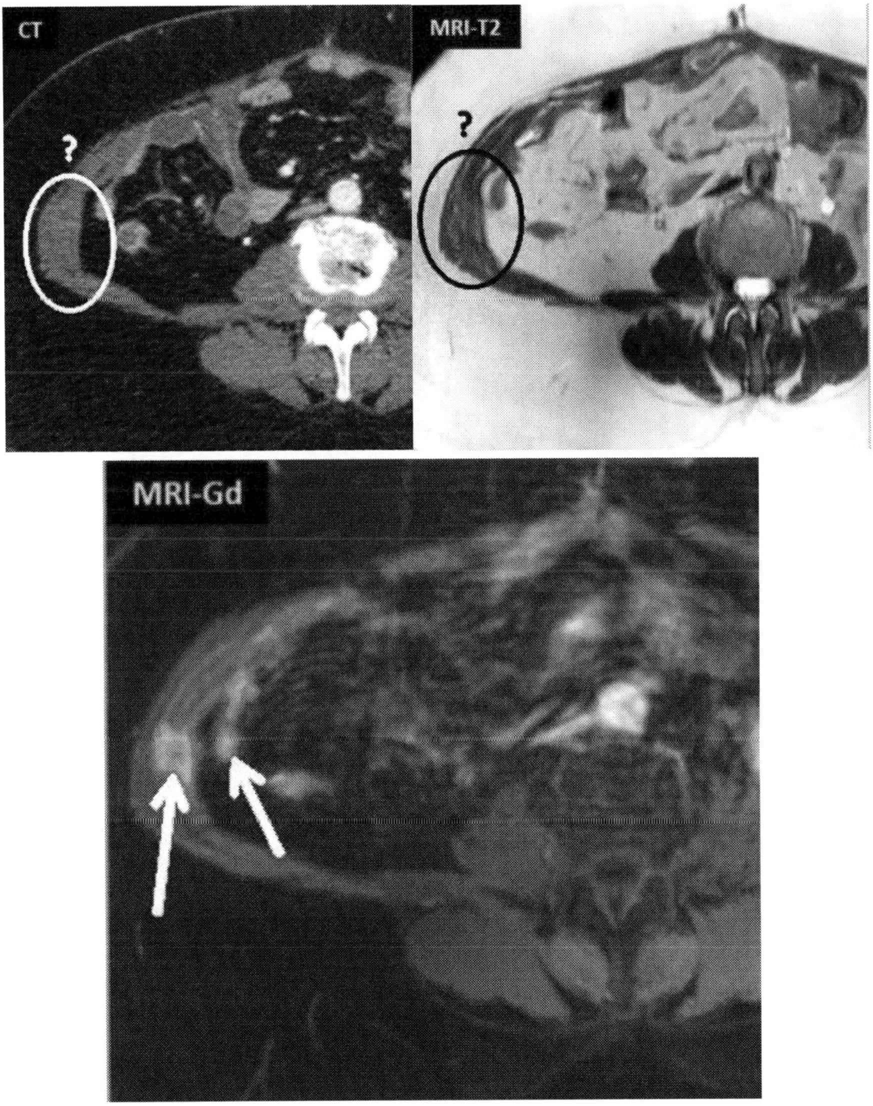

Figure 4.9. In this patient with colorectal cancer, the gadolinium-enhanced MRI displays wall infiltration of the abdominal wall. The cancer is diffusely infiltrating the muscle layers. This was only depicted on the post-contrast sequence (arrows) and not on CT or T2 images. The surgeon will be grateful if you warn him of such lesions.

Post-contrast sequences after gadolinium are also useful in two particular types of lesion. First these sequences better define mucinous lesions in pseudomyxoma peritonei. It helps to differentiate amorphous mucinous (mucinous ascites) from the mucinous tumor nodules. On CT in Figure 4.8 only ascites in the pouch of Douglas can be seen. But on MRI post-contrast sequences, you see not only amorphous ascites but also a thick enhancement of the pelvic parietal peritoneum. Second, these sequences well display abdominal wall involvement. In Figure 4.9 in a patient with colorectal cancer there is extrinsic extension from the peritoneum through the abdominal wall. Infiltration of the different muscular layers well depicted on post contrast sequence is not seen on T2 and neither on CT.

Another type of abdominal wall lesion well depicted by post-contrast MRI is disease at a laparoscopic trocar port site. Figure 4.10 shows on the left flank a nodular tumor precisely in the location of the laparoscopy trocar. While these lesions are sometimes difficult to palpate on clinical examination they are obvious on gadolinium-enhanced MRI.

Diffusion-Weighted MRI Imaging of Peritoneal Metastases

In addition to morphological sequences, functional sequences with diffusion-weighted imaging improve tumor implant detection [4, 5]. The high cellularity of peritoneal nodules results in a bright spot within a dark background making tumor nodules easier to depict. Low and colleagues nicely demonstrated that association of a combination of morphological sequences with diffusion increases the sensitivity of MRI detection of lesions by 20% [5].

As shown in Figure 4.11 two nodules in the deep part of the falciform ligament can clearly be depicted on diffusion sequence while they are also present on the morphological sequences. Diffusion MRI has to be combined with morphological sequences to avoid isolated diffusion spots and avoid false positives [6, 7].

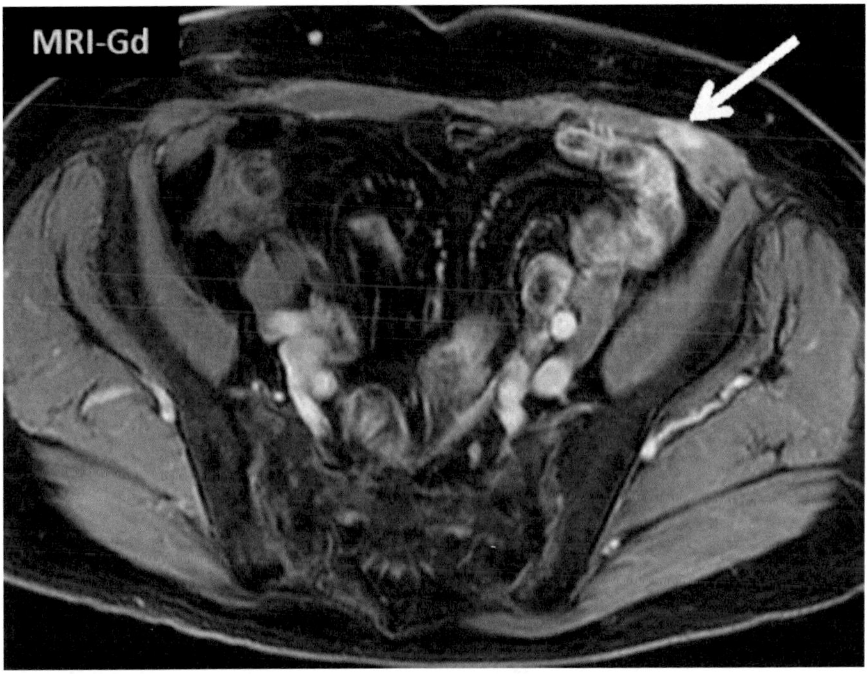

Figure 4.10. Shows a second type of abdominal wall involvement at the laparoscopy trocar site in a patient with colorectal cancer (arrow).

Diffusion-weighted imaging will also help you to depict lesions undetected on CT because the tumor nodules are isodense to the surrounding structures. In the colon cancer patient shown in Figure 4.12, the sigmoid colon lesion cannot be seen on CT while it is well depicted on diffusion-weighted MRI image.

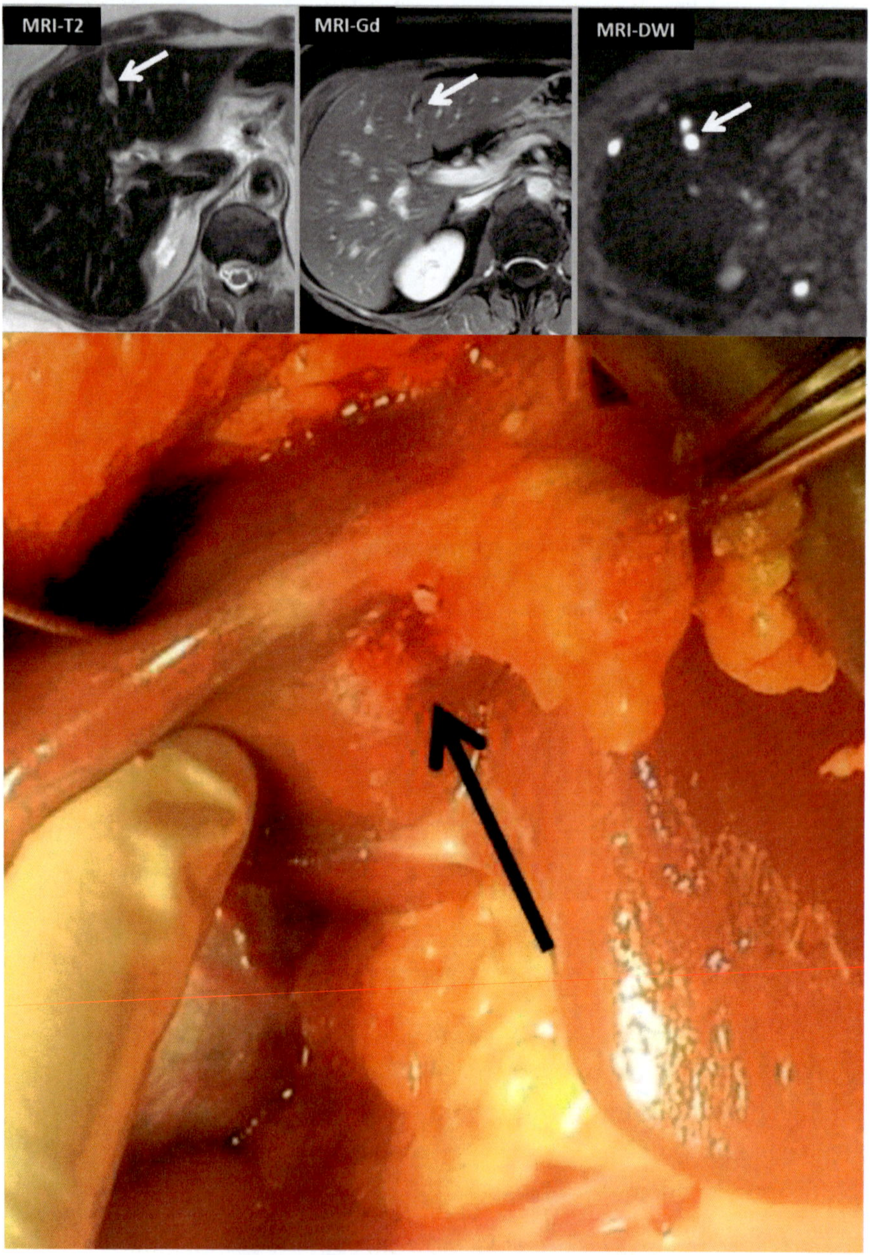

Figure 4.11. Top. In this patient with ovarian cancer, MRI displays a small deposit deep in the falciform ligament (arrows) which is easier to detect on the diffusion sequence than on T2 or post-contrast sequence. Bottom. An intraoperative photograph showing the ovarian cancer nodules on the ligaments and surface of the liver.

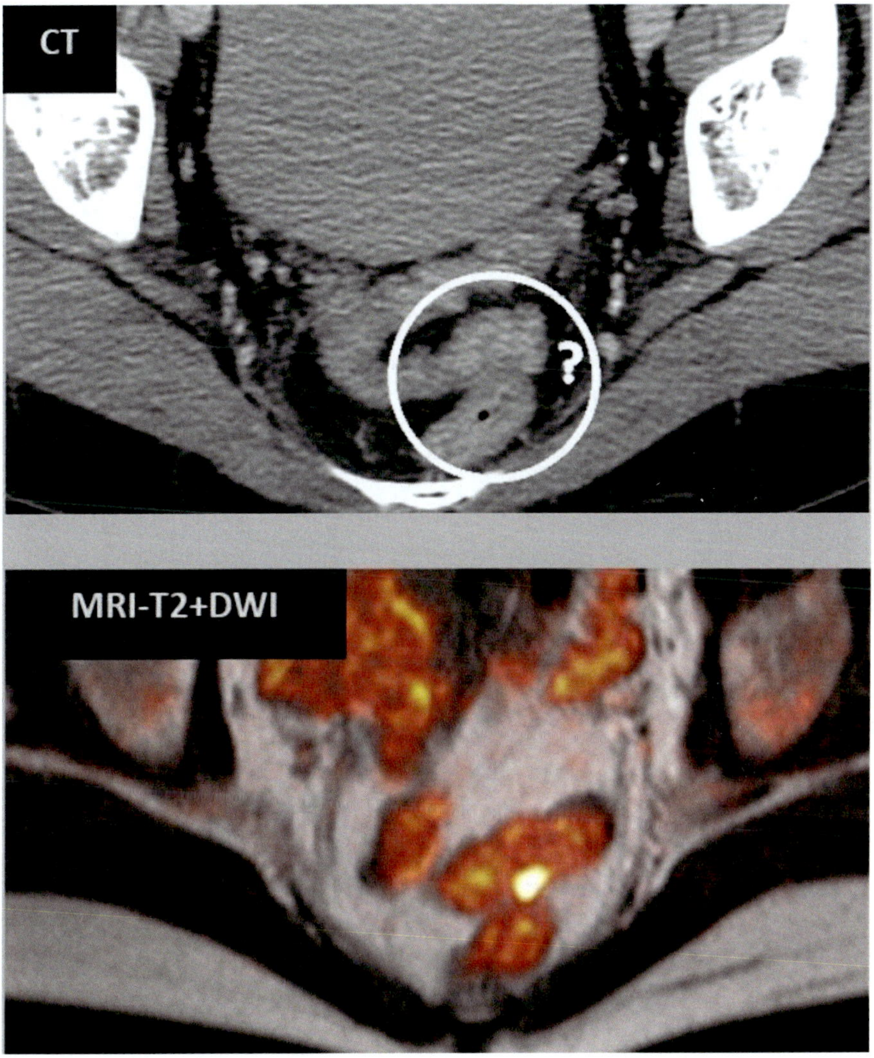

Figure 4.12. In a patient with colorectal cancer, peritoneal implant on the sigmoid colon was not depicted by CT but was appreciated by diffusion-weighted MRI fused with T2 image.

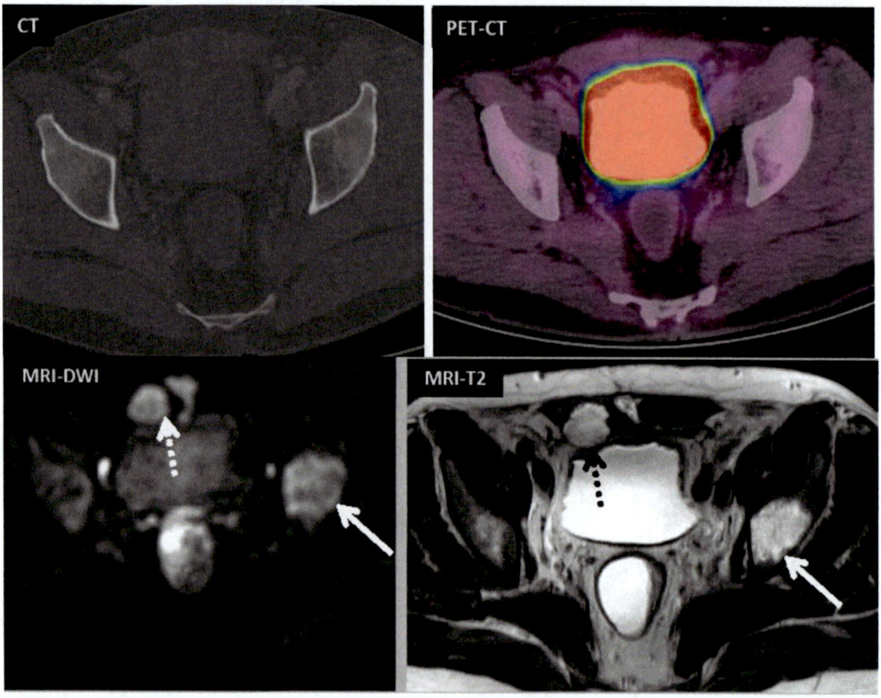

Figure 4.13. This patient followed for pseudomyxoma peritonei of urachal origin eligible for a curative surgery based on CT but also based on PET-CT with a false positive mucinous osseous lesion due to a low cellularity lesion. Diffusion-weighted images and T2-weighted sequences clearly depict an osseous lesion (arrows) which has the same pattern as the pelvic recurrence (dashed arrows).

Diffusion-weighted MRI also helps to detect extraperitoneal lesions including lymph node, liver or osseous metastases. The patient shown in Figure 4.13 was being considered for curative surgery with a recurrence of pseudomyxoma peritonei of urachal origin. MRI was very useful to prevent unnecessary surgery depicting a huge osseous lesion.

Limitations of MRI for Peritoneal Metastases

MRI has many advantages but also limitations. Some limitations are well known - the lower availability, the higher cost, and the longtime of examination are real considerations.

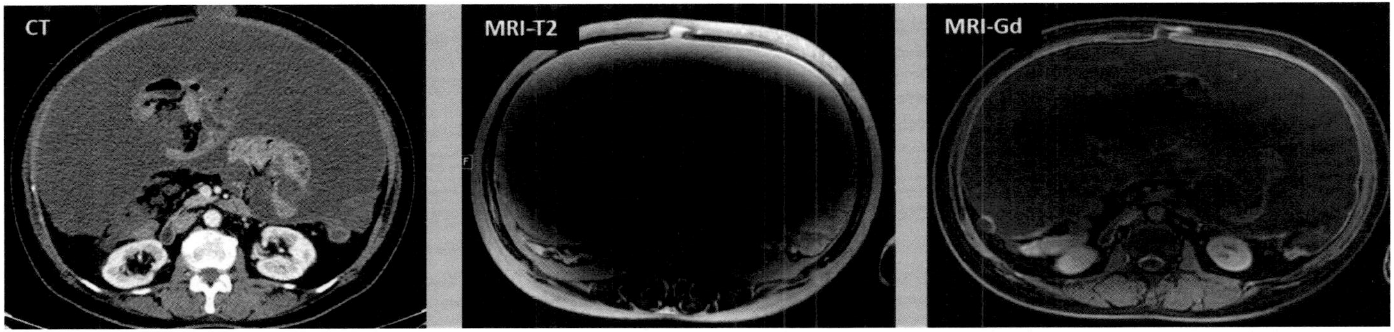

Figure 4.14. Central black hole artifact on MRI, more important on T2 than post contrast sequence, due to large amount of mucinous ascites in a patient with pseudomyxoma.

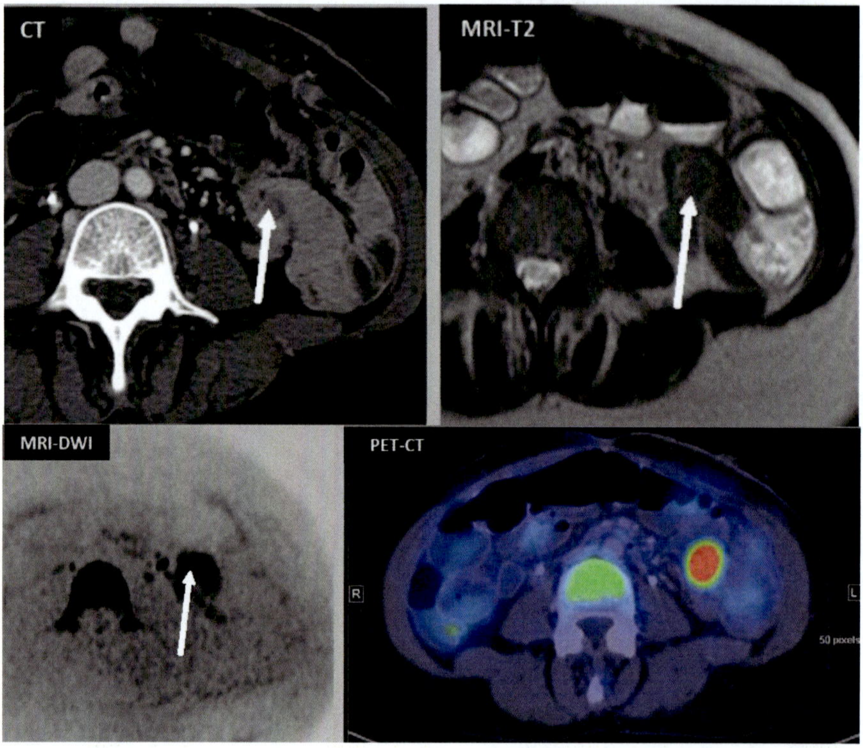

Figure 4.15. Left mesenteric lesion (arrows) better seen on PET-CT in a patient with colorectal cancer.

Some limitations depend on the patient. Motion and breathing artifacts are more frequent in debilitated patients. In some patients, at the end of the examination due to patient fatigue, respiratory-triggered sequences should be used or repetition of breath hold sequences has to be performed, but they make the examination longer. There are also bowel peristalsis artifacts, which cause blurring and alters the quality of the image. If the patient is stressed or tired, MRI may not be of benefit. Oral contrast and CT may be the preferred imaging modality. Another limitation depending on the patient is the black hole artifact due to large volume of ascites (Figure 4.14).

This artifact is more problematic on high field 3.0-T MR scanners. It is due to magnetic field loss at the central part of the ascites and technique cannot do much about this artifact. It is more likely to occur on T2 images which have a longer time of relaxation. It is more important where the ascites is more predominant, mostly at the mid-abdominal level. A paracentesis is preferred before an MRI otherwise CT should be performed.

Another limitation for the radiologist is a prolonged learning curve. The K-value on MRI is lower than on PET-CT, as when hypermetabolic lesions are easy to see (Figure 4.15).

Other limitations depend on the technique. MRI is well known to have a low spatial resolution. This is less true thanks to 3D images or Dixon images with a slice thickness of 2 or 3 mm (Figure 4.16). Diffusion-weighted MRI sequences also have limitations. Its main weakness is its lack of specificity and the risk of false positive findings. Cystic or cystic-like lesions can appear hyperintense on diffusion images due to T2 shine through effect. To minimize this effect, high b value (>800 s/mm^2) should be used, and radiologist should also read apparent diffusion coefficient (ADC) map, which eliminates the T2 component of the signal. Normal structures also have physiological restrictions and are hyperintense on diffusion-weighted MRI images such as lymph nodes, spleen, bowel submucosa (Figure 4.17). Inflammatory lesions as well as lesions with thick or hemorrhagic content more frequent after surgery can also be misleading because they are hyperintense on diffusion-weighted MRI images. In contrast, there are false negatives on diffusion-weighted images due to lesions with a low cellularity. In most cases, these lesions correspond to fat stranding on CT images and fat stranding is also difficult to depict on morphological sequences (Figure 4.18). Subtle to moderate fat stranding may be better depicted on CT. CT is superior to depict these lesions by a combination of high spatial resolution with the spontaneous high contrast of hypodense adipose tissue.

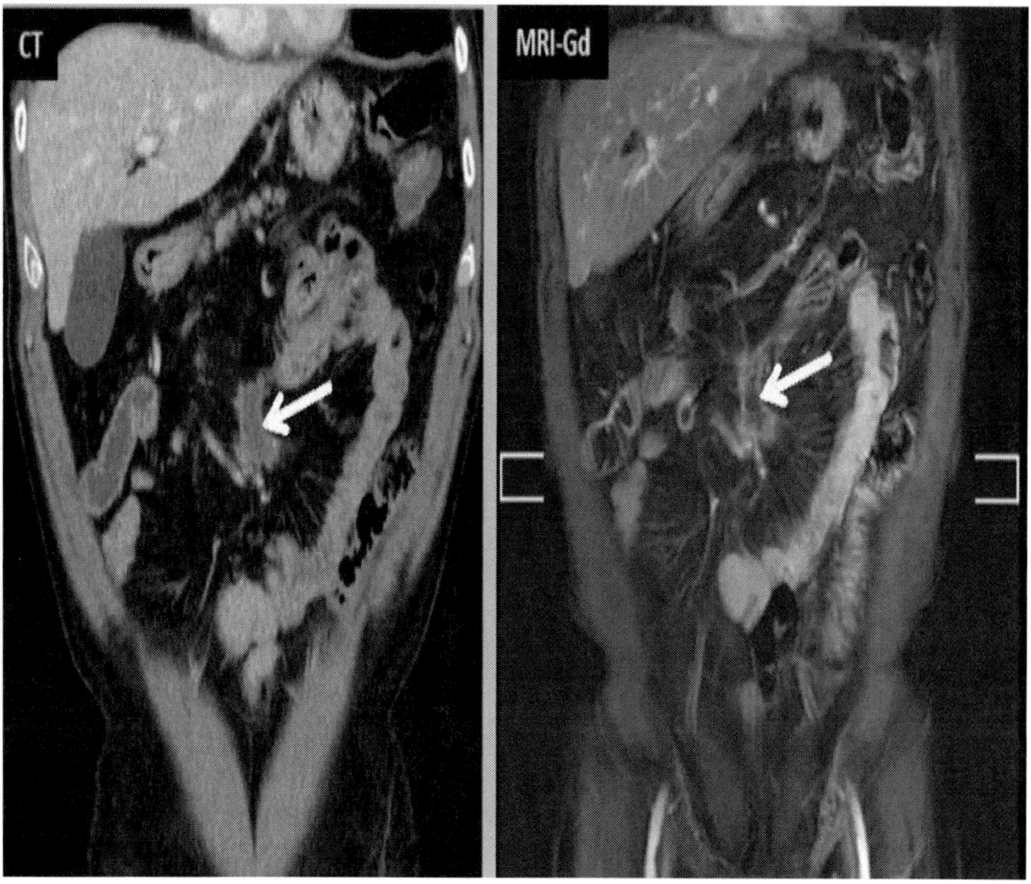

Figure 4.16. In this patient with a colorectal cancer, coronal post-contrast MRI image demonstrates a high spatial and contrast resolution that allows a precise description of the mesenteric necrotic metastases (arrows) similar to CT.

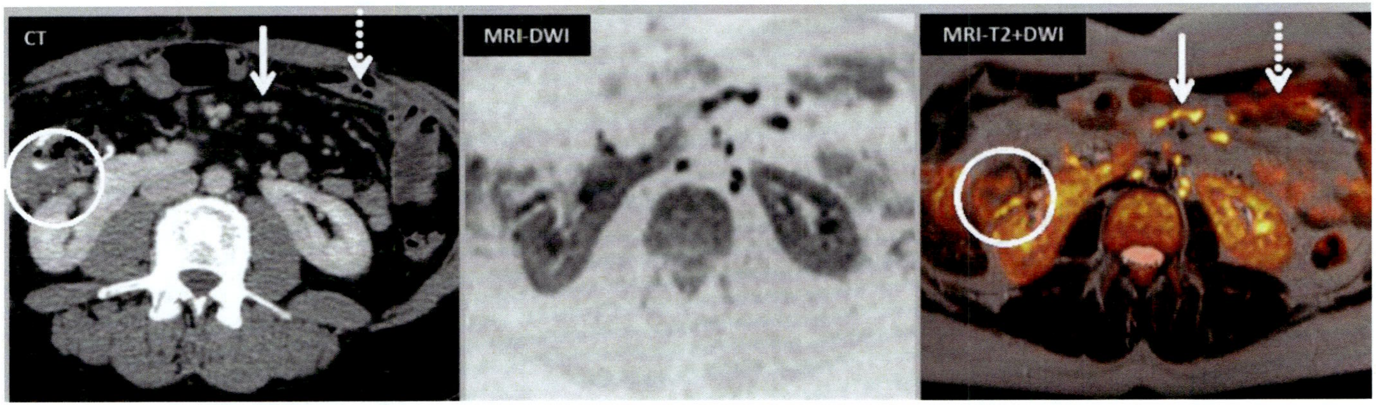

Figure 4.17. In this patient with previous colorectal cancer, the surgeon only found a recurrence on the ileocolic anastomosis in the right flank (circle) and nothing on the mesentery (arrows) or on the small bowel (dashed arrows). The hyperintense signal on diffusion images correspond to physiologic restriction in lymph nodes (arrows) and small bowel submucosae (dashed arrows).

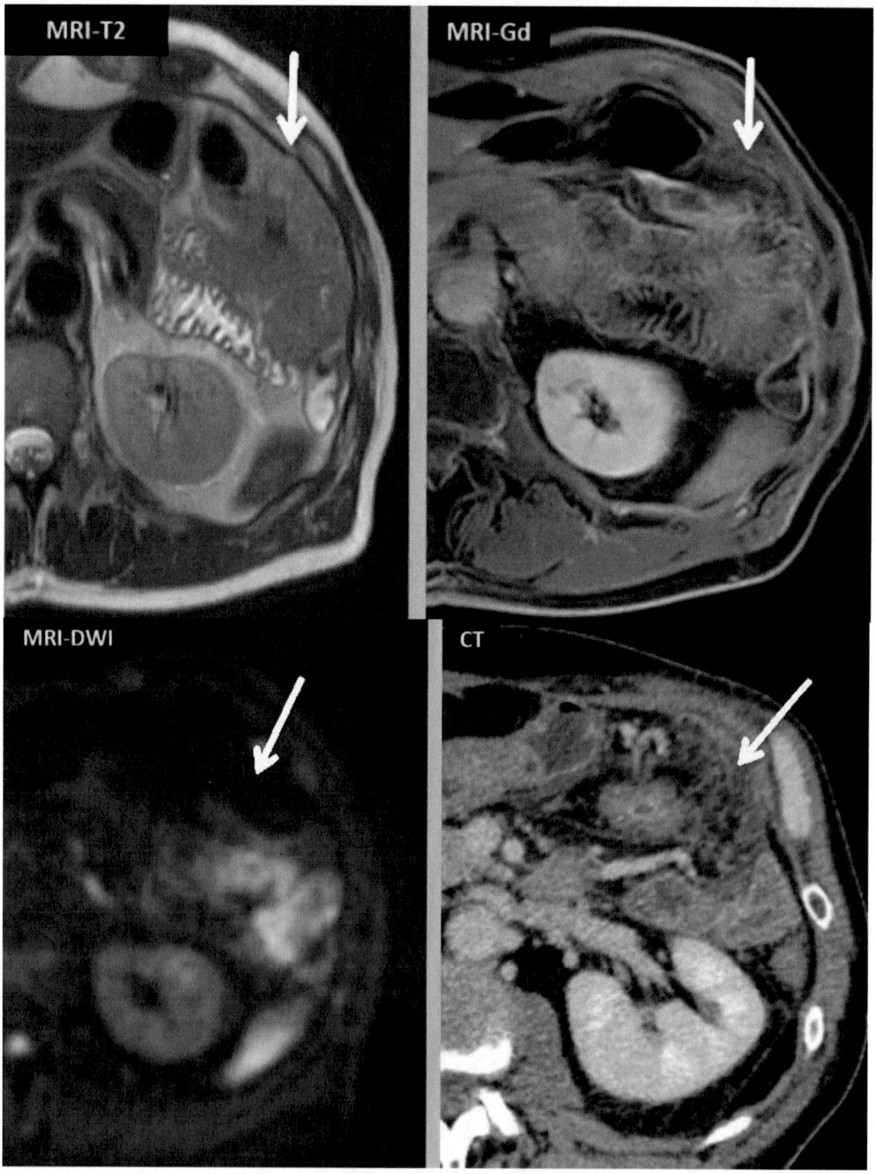

Figure 4.18. In this patient with gastric cancer, the infiltration of the left upper part of the greater omentum (arrows) is better depicted on CT compared to MRI, particularly with absence of hypersignal on diffusion image. In contrast, the diffusion-weighted images suggest jejunal serosal tumor anterior to the left kidney, which is not visible on CT.

PERFORMANCE OF PERITONEAL MRI

There are growing data, but there still have been few studies of peritoneal MRI over the last 10 years. The studies can be divided into those with a quantitative analysis using PCI and those with qualitative analysis.

Regarding radiological PCI, CT clearly underestimates the surgical PCI, particularly for small bowel regions as reported by Koh and colleagues and Chua and colleagues [8, 9]. Low et al. have published numerous studies that clearly show the superiority of MRI as compared to CT in series with mostly mucinous metastases from appendiceal cancer [5, 10]. They showed MRI peritoneal cancer index correctly categorized tumor volume compared to CT and has a high per site sensitivity particularly in bowel regions. Regarding peritoneal metastases from non-mucinous tumors, there are very few studies and they are very heterogeneous. Most studies have small number of patients. The MRI protocols are different and only some protocols are with diffusion-weighted images. Also, the standard of reference is not always surgical findings but sometimes only the follow-up imaging. So it is very difficult to have a clear idea. Nevertheless, none of these studies report the superiority of MRI as compared to PET-CT or CT to evaluate the extent of peritoneal disease [11-14]. A recent study in 49 patients with colorectal cancer (36 non-mucinous adenocarcinomas showed that MRI-PCI had a stronger correlation with surgical PCI, and accurately predicted resectable patients with a PCI < 21, with excellent intraclass correlations [15]. Finally, MRI can also be used in combination with CT to improve radiological PCI [16].

Regarding the studies with qualitative analysis that focused on unresectable lesions, there are very few studies. MRI, thanks to its high contrast resolution, is very accurate to depict involvement of the bladder and unresectable lesion of trigone [17] as well as small bowel involvement [18].

PERITONEAL METASTASES IN FOLLOW-UP

MRI is very useful in the initial staging but also in follow-up. In the young patient, MRI is radiation-free and is acceptable for serial examinations. In two studies, Low et al., demonstrate that MRI can detect recurrence, even sometimes earlier than serial tumor markers [19, 20]. Our experience is the same regarding multicystic as well as malignant mesothelioma (Figure 4.19).

In conclusion, MRI is definitely a well-established technique thanks to the high contrast resolution and technical improvements. MRI is a robust and a sensitive examination that can depict peritoneal metastases and, in some cases, it can depict lesions that are not seen with other techniques. There is growing data to suggest that MRI should be the technique of choice for pseudomyxoma peritonei and mucinous adenocarcinoma staging. In our experience it should be the same for mesothelioma. Regarding peritoneal metastases from other origins, MRI has a great potential but, nevertheless, further large multicentric studies are needed to determine the role of MRI. The next field to explore is the evaluation of tumor response after treatment. Thanks to its functional capabilities, some teams are currently evaluating apparent diffusion coefficient (ADC) and/or texture analysis as potential surrogate markers of early response and/or indicators of the disease-free survival.

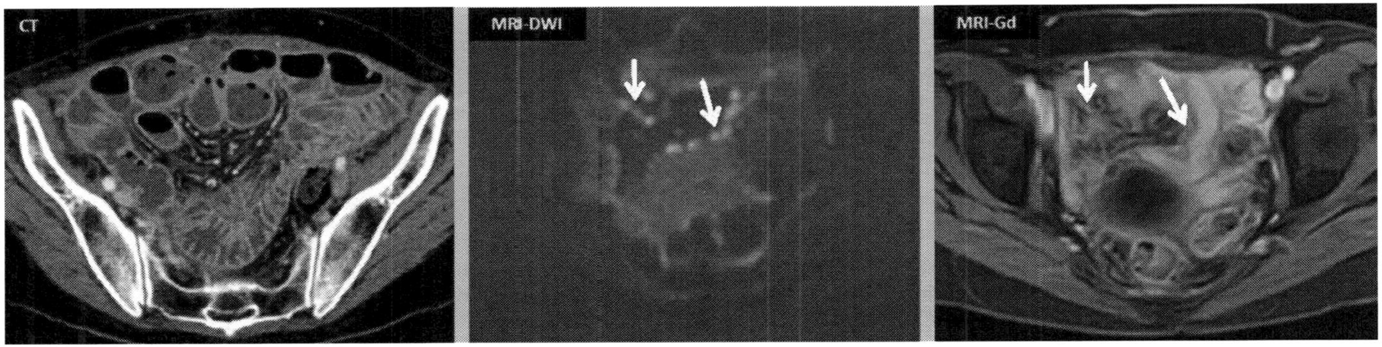

Figure 4.19. In this patient in 7 months follow-up for mesothelioma with abdominal pain, CT shows some subtle small bowel abnormalities but no clear lesion. MRI performed a few days after shows enhancement of the mesentery and nodular lesions on the small bowel serosa (arrows) that were confirmed to be tumor at surgery.

REFERENCES

[1] Low RN. MR imaging of the peritoneal spread of malignancy. *Abdom. Imaging*. 2007 May-Jun;32(3):267-83.

[2] Low RN, Barone RM. Imaging for Peritoneal Metastases. *Surg. Oncol. Clin. N Am.* 2018 Jul;27(3):425-442.

[3] Low RN. Preoperative and surveillance MR imaging of patients undergoing cytoreductive surgery and heated intraperitoneal chemotherapy. *J. Gastrointest. Oncol*. 2016 Feb;7(1):58-71.

[4] Low RN, Barone RM. Combined diffusion-weighted and gadolinium-enhanced MRI can accurately predict the peritoneal cancer index preoperatively in patients being considered for cytoreductive surgical procedures. *Ann. Surg. Oncol.* 2012 May;19(5):1394-1401.

[5] Low RN, Sebrechts CP, Barone RM, Muller W. Diffusion-weighted MRI of peritoneal tumors: comparison with conventional MRI and surgical and histopathologic findings - a feasibility study. *Am. J. Roentgenol.* 2009 Aug;193(2):461-70.

[6] Satoh Y, Ichikawa T, Motosugi U, et al. Diagnosis of peritoneal dissemination: comparison of 18F-FDG PET/CT, diffusion-weighted MRI, and contrast enhanced MDCT. *Am. J. Roentgenol.* 2011;196:447-453.

[7] Bozkurt M, Doganay S, Kantarci M, et al. Comparison of peritoneal tumor imaging using conventional MR imaging and diffusion-weighted MR imaging with different b values. *Eur. J. Radiol.* 2011;80(2):224-228.

[8] Koh JL, Yan TD, Glenn D, Morris DL. Evaluation of preoperative computed tomography in estimating peritoneal cancer index in colorectal peritoneal carcinomatosis. *Ann. Surg. Oncol*. 2009;16:327-333.

[9] Chua TC, Al-Zahrani A, Saxena A, et al. Determining the association between preoperative computed tomography findings and post-operative outcomes after cytoreductive surgery and perioperative

intraperitoneal chemotherapy for pseudomyxoma peritonei. *Ann. Surg. Oncol.* 2011;18(6):1582-1589.

[10] Low RN, Barone RM, Lucero J. Comparison of MRI and CT for predicting the Peritoneal Cancer Index (PCI) preoperatively in patients being considered for cytoreductive surgical procedures. *Ann. Surg. Oncol.* 2015 May;22(5):1708-15.

[11] Qayyum A, Coakley FV, Westphalen AC, et al. Role of CT and MR imaging in predicting optimal cytoreduction of newly diagnosed primary epithelial ovarian cancer. *Gynecol. Oncol.* 2005;96(2):301-306.

[12] Torkzad MR, Casta N, Bergman A, et al. Comparison between MRI and CT in prediction of peritoneal carcinomatosis index (PCI) in patients undergoing cytoreductive surgery in relation to the experience of the radiologist. *J. Surg. Oncol.* 2015;111(6):746-751.

[13] Soussan M, Des Guetz G, Barrau V, et al. Comparison of FDG-PET/CT and MR with diffusion-weighted imaging for assessing peritoneal carcinomatosis from gastrointestinal malignancy. *Eur. Radiol.* 2012;22(7):1479-1487.

[14] Klumpp BD, Aschoff P, Schwenzer N, et al. Peritoneal carcinomatosis: comparison of dynamic contrast-enhanced magnetic resonance imaging with surgical and histopathologic findings. *Abdom. Imaging.* 2012;37(5):834-842.

[15] Van't Sant I, van Eden WJ, Engbersen MP, Kok NFM, Woensdregt K, Lambregts DMJ, Shanmuganathan S, Beets-Tan RGH, Aalbers AGJ, Lahaye MJ. Diffusion-weighted MRI assessment of the peritoneal cancer index before cytoreductive surgery. *Br. J. Surg.* 2018 Oct 24. https://doi.org/10.1002/bjs.10989.

[16] Dohan A, Hoeffel C, Soyer P, et al. Evaluation of the peritoneal carcinomatosis index with CT and MRI. *Br. J. Surg.* Aug 2017;104(9):1244-1249.

[17] Cotton F, Pellet O, Gilly FN, Granier A, Sournac L, Glehen O. MRI evaluation of bulky tumor masses in the mesentery and bladder involvement in peritoneal carcinomatosis. *Eur. J. Surg. Oncol.* 2006;32:1212-1216.

[18] Menassel B, Duclos A, Passot G, Dohan A, Payet C, Isaac S, Valette PJ, Glehen O, Rousset P. Preoperative CT and MRI prediction of non-respectability in patients treated for pseudomyxoma peritonei from mucinous appendiceal neoplasms. *Eur. J. Surg. Oncol.* 2016 Apr;42(4):558-66.

[19] Low RN, Duggan B, Barone RM, Saleh F, Song SY. Treated ovarian cancer: MR imaging, laparotomy reassessment, and serum CA-125 values compared with clinical outcome at 1 year. *Radiology.* 2005;235:918-926.

[20] Low RN, Barone RM, Lee MJ. Surveillance MR imaging is superior to serum tumor markers for detecting early tumor recurrence in patients with appendiceal cancer treated with surgical cytoreduction and HIPEC. *Ann. Surg. Oncol.* 2013 Apr;20(4):1074-81.

In: Pictorial Essays … ISBN: 978-1-53618-014-5
Editors: PH Sugarbaker and RN Low ©2020 Nova Science Publishers, Inc.

Chapter 5

RADIOLOGIC DESCRIPTION AND INTERPRETATION OF PATTERNS OF RECURRENCE OF RECTAL CANCER

Gina Brown, MD
Royal Marsden and Imperial College, London, UK

INTRODUCTION

The goal for this presentation is to describe radiologically the patterns of failure of rectal cancer surgery, to assist in understanding the causation of disease recurrence and to offer modification of standard treatments to be able to prevent recurrence disease. The challenge is to figure out why our pre- and intraoperative treatments of rectal cancer were inadequate. Often, the Peritoneal Surface Oncology Group surgeon is the one asked to attempt salvage of these recurrences. However, the more far reaching question is "How did the clinical situation get to this position so that salvage is necessary?" One outcome of this critique may be to identify those patients who needed but did not receive adequate preoperative or intraoperative therapy.

One of the huge misconceptions in colorectal cancer management is the belief that progression of disease in lymph nodes is responsible for the recurrences. I am unable to rationalize how lymph nodal disease will cause the patterns of recurrence that we see. It is not possible! We do know that peritoneal spread will progress to pelvic recurrence. We do know that vascular invasion can cause recurrence from seeding to the pelvic sidewall compartments. We do know that margin-positive disease or a badly performed total mesorectal excision (TME) will eventuate in disease progression at a predetermined site [1]. Progression within lymph nodes does not explain recurrent disease! Yet lymph nodal progression as a prominent cause of surgical treatment failure is enshrined in oncological thinking.

Something is misaligned here, and treatment failures need to be forensically studied. Currently, I am convinced we lack the necessary precision to identify the culprit in recurrent disease in rectal cancer. Is it surgical treatment failure due to faulty primary surgery? Alternatively, is it due to an advanced tumor having breached the mesorectal fascia? Might it have to do with inadequate investigation of the primary cancer with undertreatment of the tumor preoperatively? Perhaps it is not due to the limitations of the technique of the primary surgery, because currently we don't know how to do it better. These possibilities really need to be looked at forensically. Currently, a lot of time and money is being invested by pharma to seek answers to clinical situations that may be completely irrelevant. The cause of treatment failure and its effect in terms of anatomic sites of recurrent disease need to be identified. A lot of the genetic work and search for actionable gene profiles may be a misguided approach, because the mechanisms for recurrence are mechanical and anatomic, not genetic. My thinking and all the radiologic evidence points in that direction. As a radiologist who sees a lot of recurrences, I am convinced we need to think not how to best treat recurrence, but also how to devise new approaches for prevention of recurrences with improved management strategies of the primary rectal cancer.

Radiologic Patterns of Recurrence of Rectal Cancer

As I compare preoperative and postoperative radiologic studies, I see predictable patterns of recurrence. These cause and effect relationships apply not just in the lower gastrointestinal area, which is my main area of interest, but also with upper gastrointestinal disease. There are 5 major causes for recurrent rectal cancer: tumor spillage, circumferential radial margin (CRM) involvement, peritoneal perforation, distal margin involvement, and incomplete resections. All 5 causes result in macro- or microscopic residual disease. When I identify a recurrence radiologically, I attempt to identify the cause. It may be one of these patterns or a mixture, but the cause will generally be included within the list provided in Table 5.1. Anastomotic recurrence must be due to tumor spillage, and that is independent of the original tumor stage. This may be due to faulty stapling technique or to an unfortunate event during the stapling procedure. CRM involvement may be due to understaging by the original radiologic imaging so that the surgeon ended up producing a positive margin when they should have had a "Beyond TME approach." Peritoneal perforation will manifest itself as peritoneal recess recurrences. Distal margin involvement will produce a perineal or peri-anastomotic recurrence. Residual disease due to incomplete TME will be obvious on your scan. For rectal cancer, these patterns of surgical treatment failure can be documented radiologically when they are first clinically apparent and often even before symptoms occur.

Table 5.1. Radiologically defined dissemination of rectal cancer

Tumor spillage
Circumferential Radial Margin (CRM) involvement
Peritoneal perforation
Distal margin involvement
Incomplete resection causing residual disease
Lymph nodal progression rarely occurs.

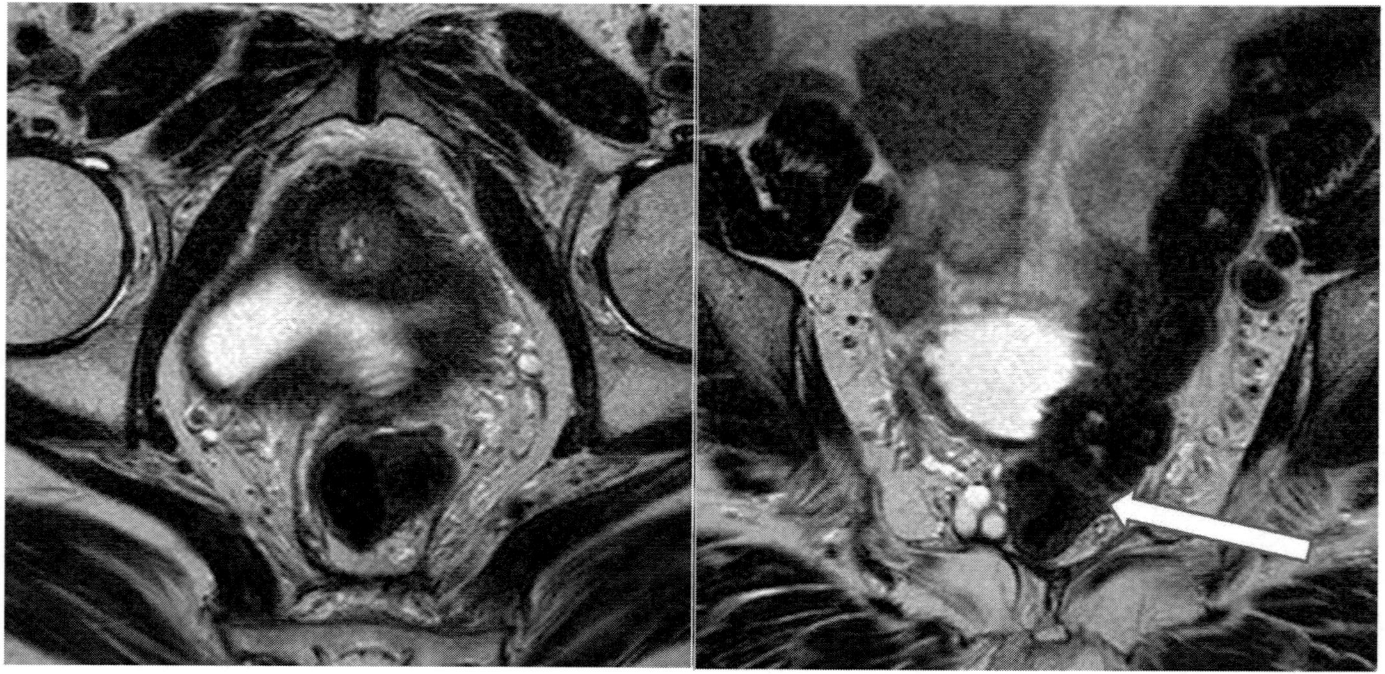

Figure 5.1. Radiologic appearance by MRI of a postsurgical pelvis. There has been a clean resection of a rectal cancer. The linear scar at the anastomotic site is indicated by the arrow

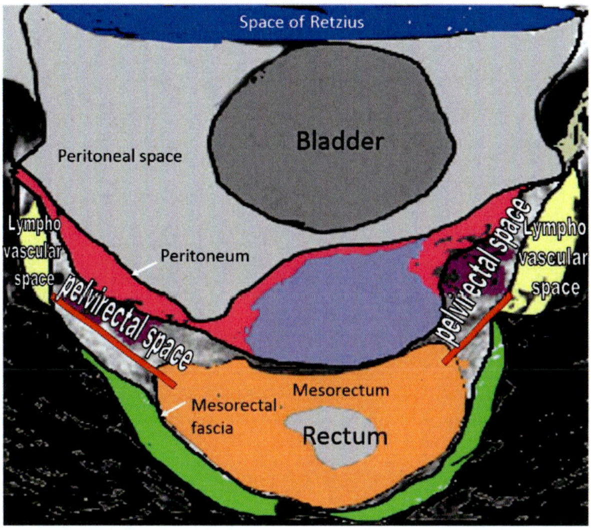

Figure 5.2. Radiologic compartments of the pelvis after a total mesorectal excision.

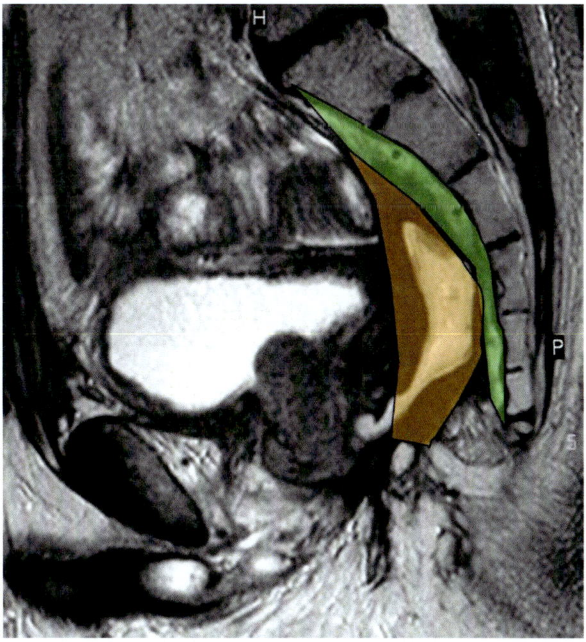

Figure 5.3. Pelvic MRI showing fluid in the lower pelvis (shaded brown) anterior to the presacral space (shaded green). Care must be taken at nodular sites of recurrent disease that may be obscured by the ascites.

Radiologically, the post-surgical pelvis should appear similar to Figure 5.1. It should look neat and tidy with a linear scar at the anastomosis. Tissues should not be thickened, nor inflamed, and should not exhibit intermediate signal intensity. This is what a post-surgical pelvis should look like after proper clearance and containment of the malignancy. If you are not seeing these post-operative images routinely from your referral centers, questions need to be asked about the primary surgical technique.

Figure 5.2 shows the compartments to identify radiologically after a TME. The diagram allows one to identify where recurrences are anatomically located, from where they are originating, and to generate a hypothesis regarding the etiology of recurrence. So, for example, lymph nodes do not occur in the pelvi-rectal space. So, if you are seeing a tumor mass in that space, then it got there either through peritoneal seeding or through vascular spread. The vessels will be traversing laterally from the mesorectum to the pelvic sidewall compartment. Venous invasion may be responsible for tumor spread by dissection in the space between the lateral pelvic sidewall fascia and the mesorectal compartment. Radiologic anatomy can be used to figure out the mechanisms of disease recurrence. Also, using this diagram is a convenient way to survey the compartments, because you can go through them systematically as you review them to detect pelvic recurrent disease.

Figure 5.3 shows a post-surgical pelvis. It is not ideal for radiological interpretation because the lower pelvic cavity is filled with fluid. This makes it difficult to identify sites of the recurrence. This is when you need a baseline study and serial imaging. By comparing baseline and subsequent studies, recurrent disease will be recognized. Also, administering intravenous contrast in this situation doesn't really help because everything enhances in the post-operative setting. This is not a reliable way to detect recurrences. In addition, performing a PET-CT doesn't really help because in the post-operative setting the surgical bed is PET avid and "lights up." So, if you want to identify early recurrence, you carefully examine the postoperative baseline scan compared to the post-treatment scans where the recurrence will show up in a nodular pattern. With this approach, you will see it, and it is very distinctive.

The MRI slice in Figure 5.4 shows recurrent disease that is predictable after CRM involvement. This is a very characteristic "rind-like" pattern of recurrence which is entirely preventable by a proper surgical technology at the time of the rectal cancer resection.

Figure 5.5 is an MRI slice that shows a marginal recurrence indicated by the black arrow. This pattern results either from CRM involvement or spread from vascular invasion. There are no lymph nodes in this particular area in the corner of the pelvis. Lymph node progression will occur in the space shown by the white arrow if it is going to develop.

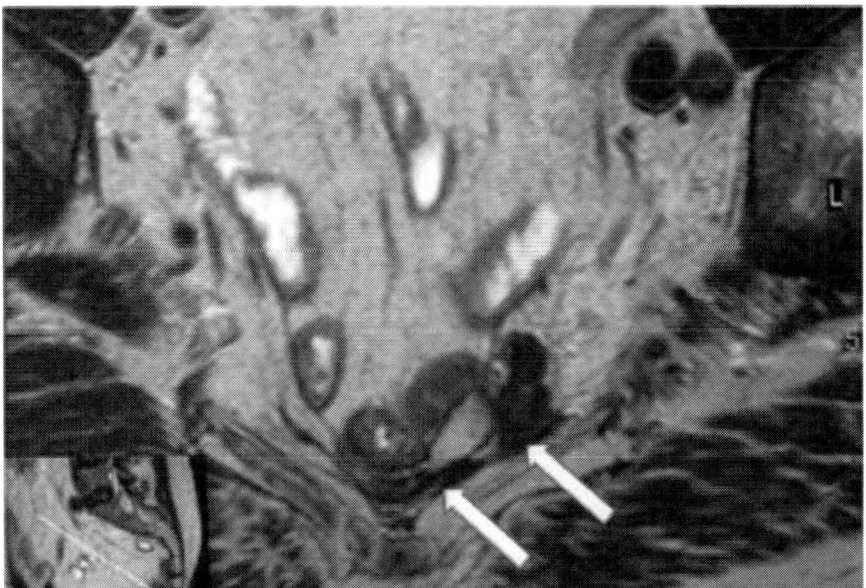

Figure 5.4. MRI of a pararectal recurrence has a "rind-like" pattern. This occurs when there is cancer cell spillage from circumferential radial margin involvement.

Figure 5.6 shows an anastomotic recurrence after a low rectal resection. Recurrent disease is at the lower aspect of the seminal vesicles.

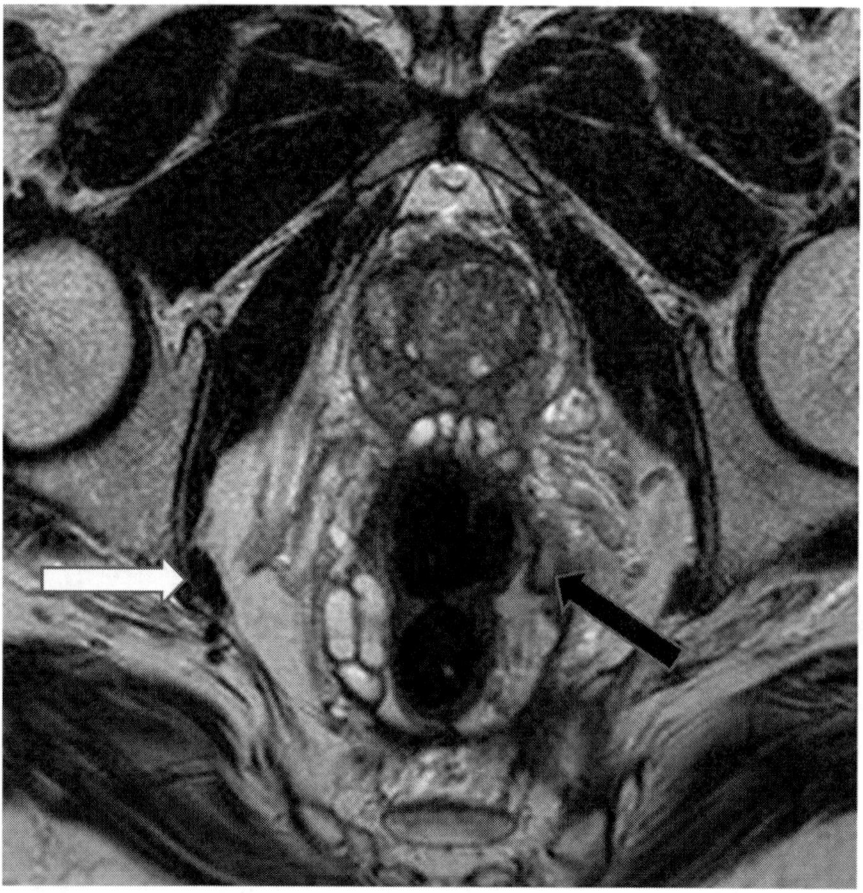

Figure 5.5. MRI slice showing a recurrence at the margin of resection indicated by the black arrow. If lymph node progression were to occur, it would be in the space shown by the white arrow.

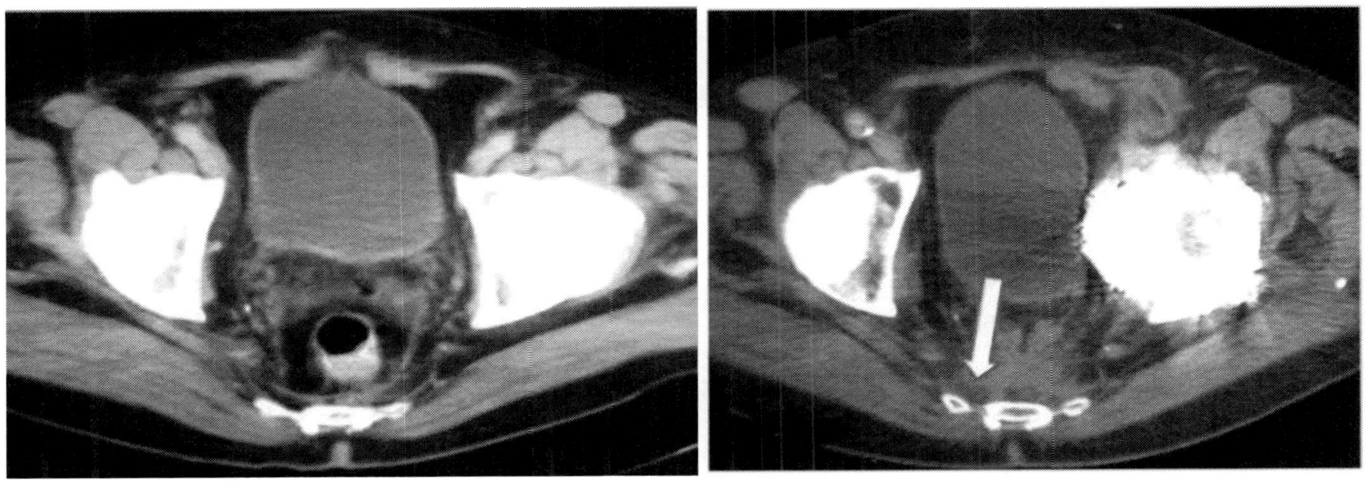

Figure 5.6. CT showing a recurrence low in the pelvis following a low rectal resection with low anastomosis.

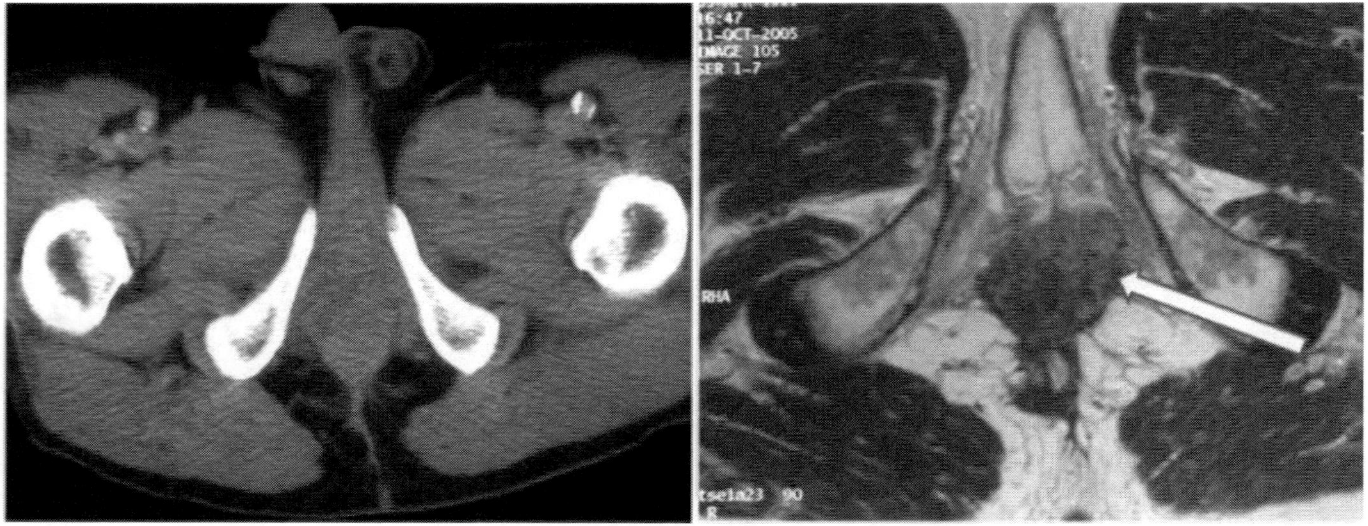

Figure 5.7. Perineal recurrence in the perineal resection site as a result of tumor spillage. CT (left) and MRI (right) slices are shown.

Figure 5.7 shows a perineal recurrence following an abdominal perineal resection. This pattern of progression was frequent before surgeons were staging low rectal cancers and using the Mercury system [2]. In the past, this was occurring in about 30-40% of patients with low rectal cancers but that has been greatly reduced. This radiologic pattern of recurrence in the perineal operative site is from tumor spillage occurring during resection (lack of containment).

One observation made a while ago concerned new onset hydroureter and hydronephrosis. If you see an unexplained dilated ureter carefully consider that this may be a manifestation of a peritoneal metastasis. The best way to sort it out is to do an MRI with high resolution through the point of obstruction of the ureter. Study carefully the distal portion of the dilated ureter. I have observed 8 times out of 10 a small peritoneal nodule causing ureteral obstruction. It is a situation that can be dealt with surgically with some long-term success.

On the left side of Figure 5.8 an unexplained right-sided hydroureter is demonstrated in a patient on follow-up CT scan. In fact, it is not just the hydroureter. In a lower cut of the CT (Figure 5.8, right), one sees peritoneal nodules infiltrating the walls of the right ureter and this is the culprit. This peritoneal disease is centered on that pelvi-rectal space and is invading into the lateral fascia. It has gone through the lateral fascia in the space where you cannot find lymph nodes. So, this is invasive peritoneal metastases that has manifested itself as ureteral obstruction. Hopefully, further scanning will reveal the extent of the disease and determine if surgical resection will benefit the patient.

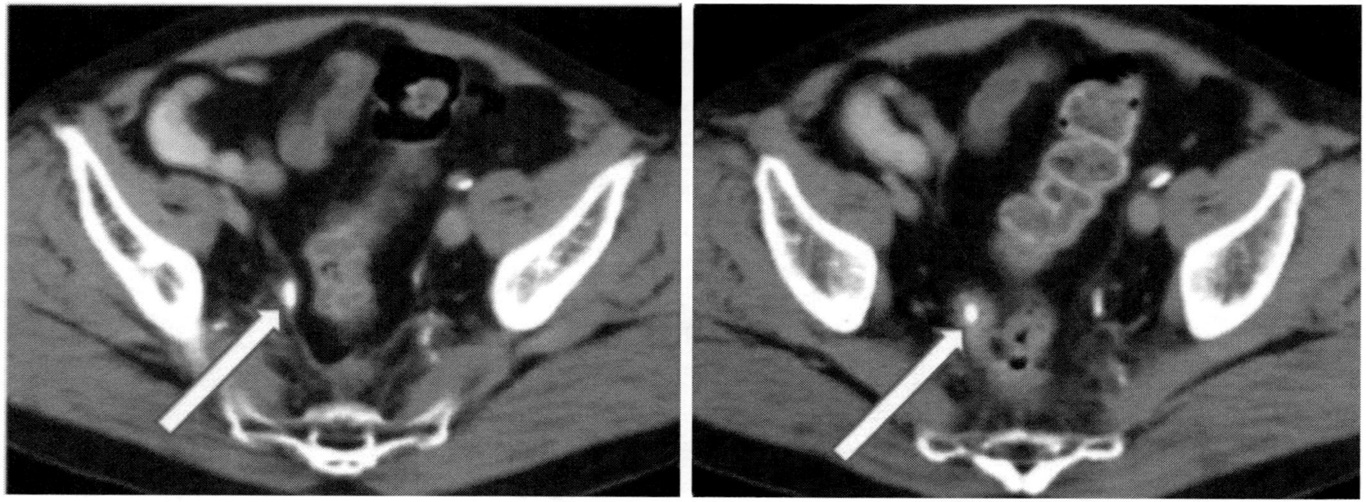

Figure 5.8 left. New onset right-sided hydroureter. Figure 5.8 right shows hydroureter caused by a localized obstruction of the lower ureter by a peritoneal metastasis. CT slices are shown.

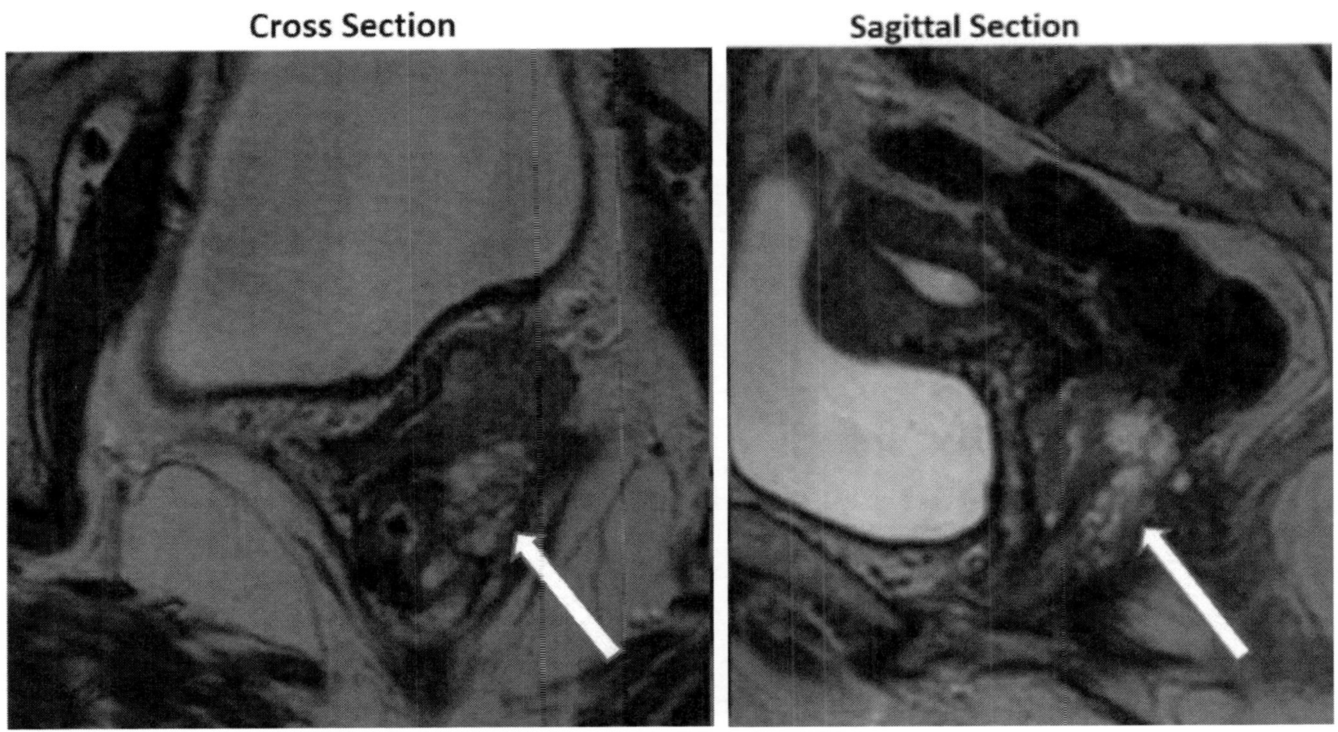

Figure 5.9. MRI axial section and sagittal section showing recurrence isolated to the distal aspect of the colorectal anastomosis.

Figure 5.9 MRI shows the distal rectal margin involved by progressive disease. This pattern will manifest itself as tumor recurring in the remnant of whatever was left behind at the distal extent of the TME. It will not be in the proximal colon but is entirely below the anastomosis. It indicates an inadequate distal margin of resection.

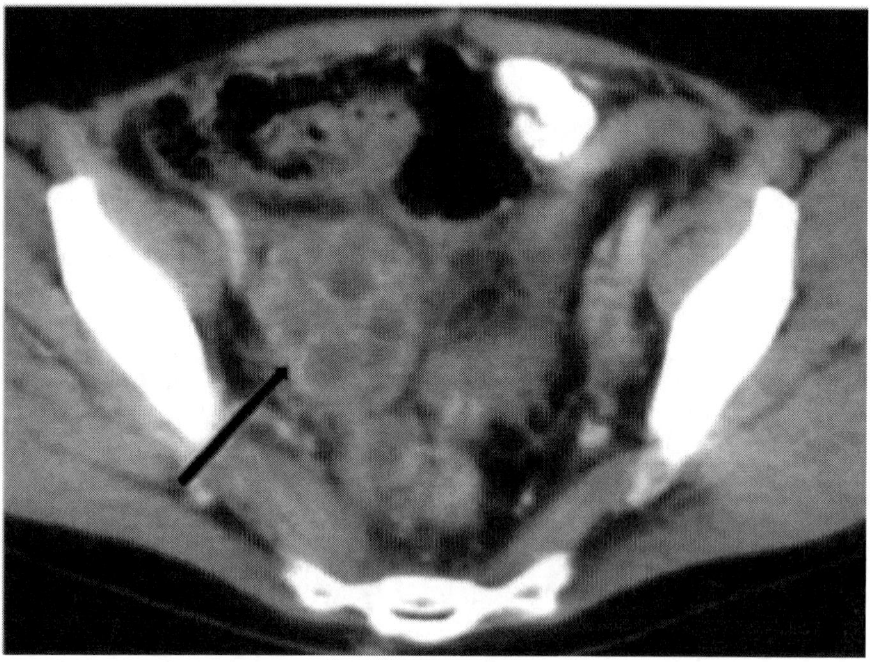

Figure 5.10. CT slice of a Krukenberg ovarian metastasis.

Figure 5.10 is a CT slice showing a Krukenberg tumor. This is an unusual but certainly not rare manifestation of peritoneal dissemination. It is from free peritoneal cancer cells and transperitoneal implantation into the ovary. Krukenberg tumors are often amenable to resection, if other sites of peritoneal metastases are limited.

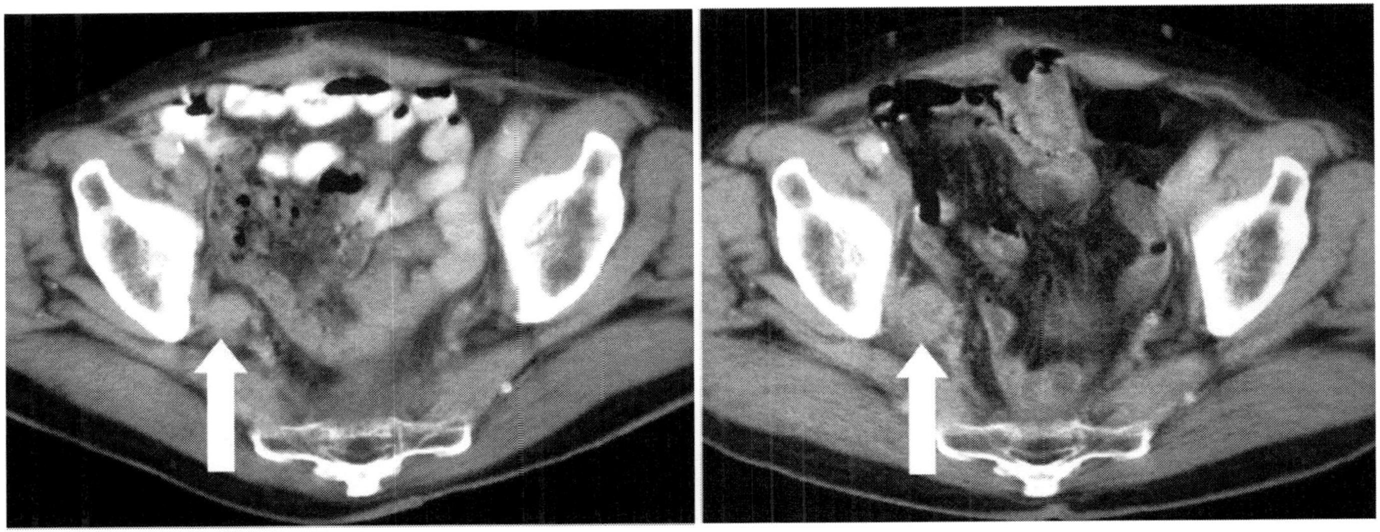

Figure 5.11. CT slices of a lymph nodal recurrence in the right lateral pelvic compartment.

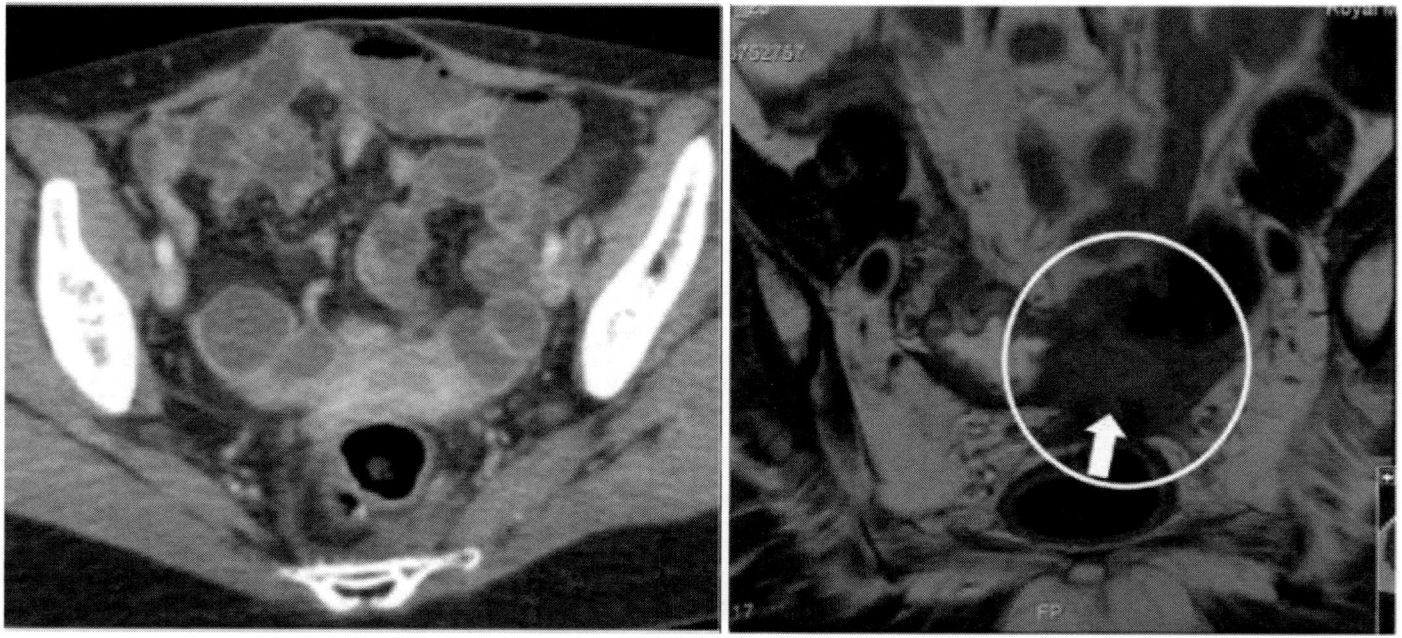

Figure 5.12. left. A CT through perirectal tissue missed the diagnosis of recurrence. PET-CT was also negative. The MRI shown in Figure 5.12. right definitively identified a recurrence within perirectal tissue that had been thought to be a bowel loop fixed in the pelvis.

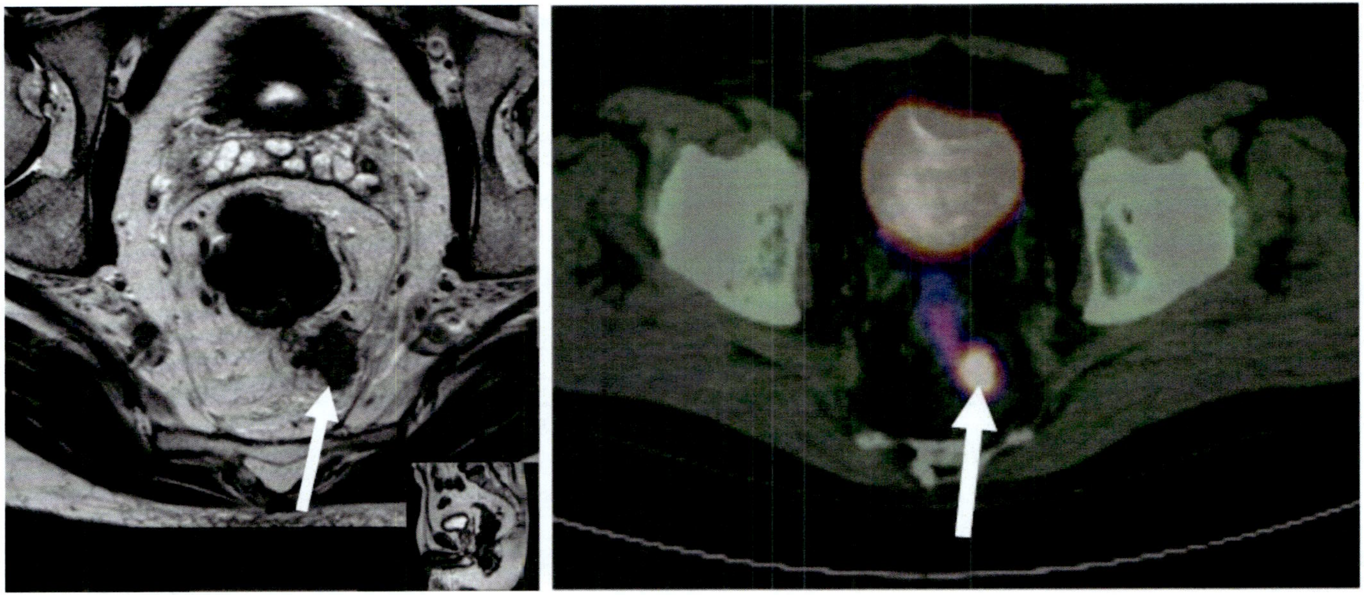

Figure 5.13. MRI (left) and PET-CT (right) show a recurrence in the perirectal fat indicating an inadequate total mesorectal excision.

Lymph nodal recurrence is unusual, but it may occur laterally. Figure 5.11 shows an example of recurrence in the pelvic sidewall compartment. Fortunately, we now have more knowledgeable use of preoperative chemoradiotherapy or postoperative radiotherapy in patients with high risk disease like extramural vascular invasion (EMVI). The risk of lateral spread has been reduced, and these late relapses of vascular-mediated nodal spread in the pelvic sidewall compartment has decreased. Vascular-mediated nodal spread may be the main route by which these tumors will reach the lateral pelvic compartment [3].

The recurrent disease in the perirectal tissue is very easy to miss. This is because it is disguised in a mass of bowel loops in the pelvis. This recurrent tumor was missed on the CT scan. The PET-CT was also negative but the CEA was rising and the patient previously had a T4 upper rectal cancer. It was very logical to image the pelvis with MRI, which confirmed definite peritoneal relapse (Figure 5.12). It was a predictable pattern of treatment failure for a patient with cancer dissemination that occurred at the time of resection of the T4 disease. Even minor surgical trauma to a T4 cancer may result in local contamination with cancer cells.

Figure 5.13 shows an example of perirectal recurrence as a result of vascular invasion. Although somewhat nodular, this is not a lymph node. It is extending out on a pedicle and is a highly vascular cancer nodule. This never started out as a lymph node. This is a discontinuous EMVI that was left in the remnant mesorectum. You can see that not much of the mesorectum was removed. This patient would have had a better outcome if he had a proper TME operation and not a partial TME. The MRI shows discontinuous vascular invasion that has recurred within an irradiated TME.

In Figure 5.14, the MRI shows recurrent cancer widely distributed within the operative sites. The tumor is occurring at the margins of the resection. These nodules of recurrent cancer are the result of tumor spillage during the operation.

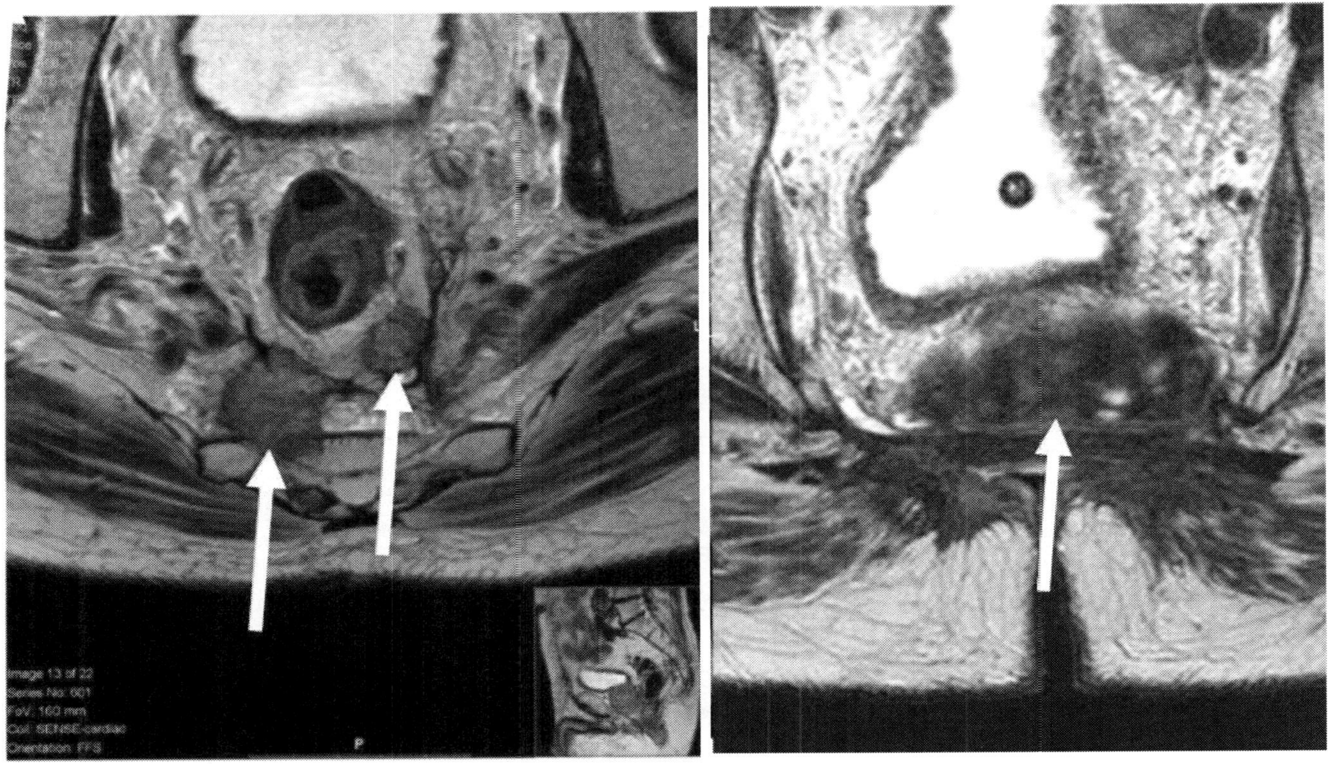

Figure 5.14. MRI in follow-up after a low rectal resection with anastomosis. The widespread disease at the resection site indicates tumor spillage with resection.

Table 5.2. Key messages to interpret radiologically rectal and sigmoid colon cancer recurrence

Know patterns of recurrence
Familiarity with post-surgical pelvis
FDG PET-CT is a helpful tool
Growing mass on CT/MRI with elevated CEA = diagnostic of recurrence, biopsy not required.

A summary of my thoughts on colorectal cancer recurrence is shown in Table 5.2. Knowing the patterns of recurrence, being familiar with the post-surgical abdomen and pelvis, FDG-PET is helpful but a growing mass in the abdomen together with an elevated CEA is pretty much diagnostic of recurrence. In my opinion it is not essential to perform a dangerous biopsy when you have this triad of abnormalities.

Aggressive imaging-based follow-up of the high-risk patients will be the way forward to improving survival. If you detect recurrences earlier, these patients are going to be more available for successful treatments at experienced centers. The anatomic description and characterization of these lesions is best done using PET-CT or MRI when multidetector CT is not positive. Consider a targeted study of the pelvis or liver depending on the original tumor stage. Finally, PET, as it is the most expensive modality, is the last choice.

I think there are some things that can be done by the Peritoneal Surface Oncology Group International which will help globally. First, start a forensic examination of the referrals that you get with recurrence. Try to track recurrence back to the primary disease because that information will be valuable for everybody in the multidisciplinary team that deals with these cancers. We do need to improve the radiologic description of tumors at baseline and compare this assessment against outcome. Secondly, there needs to be an education of the referral centers concerning what recurrent disease is resectable and what is not. So, the use of a radiologic pro-forma is the key, because at least then you can check whether you agree or not with the assessment of the referring institution. Will you have to repeat the whole radiologic workup? For the heavily-burdened central referral centers, pro-formas are essential. If you make this a condition of being referred, they must make an attempt to construct a pro-forma. This will reduce your work, and perhaps you can selectively adjust some of the other radiologic parameters.

There are definitely important considerations for assessing resectability of recurrent rectal cancer which, I think, applies to all cancer. However, in rectal cancer, the key considerations are the sacral level, the number of compartments involved, whether it is multifocal versus unifocal disease and whether or not there are distant sites of disease. Increasingly, there is a greater interest in giving these patients chemotherapy up front, more as a way of determining the biology and the natural progression of the disease [4]. If they don't respond to chemotherapy or if they progress on chemotherapy, then these patients, in our center, don't proceed to radical exenterative type surgery.

REFERENCES

[1] Quirke P., Durdey P., Dixon M. F., et al., Local recurrence of rectal adenocarcinoma due to inadequate surgical resection: histopathological study of lateral tumour spread and surgical excision. *Lancet* 1986; 2:996-999.

[2] MERCURY Study Group. Diagnostic accuracy of preoperative magnetic resonance imaging in predicting curative resection of rectal cancer: prospective observational study. *BMJ* 2006; 333:779.

[3] Chand M., Bhangu A., Wotherspoon A., et al., EMVI-positive stage II rectal cancer has similar clinical outcomes as stage III disease following pre-operative chemoradiotherapy. *Ann Oncol* 2014; 25(4):858-863.

[4] Foxtrot Collaborative Group. Feasibility of preoperative chemotherapy for locally advanced, operable colon cancer: the pilot phase of a randomised controlled trial. *Lancet Oncol* 2012; 13(11):1152-1160.

[5] Dighe S., Blake H., Koh M. D., Swift I., Arnaout A., Temple L., Barbachano Y., Brown G. Accuracy of multidetector computed tomography in identifying poor prognostic factors in colonic cancer. *Br J Surg* 2010; 97:1407-1415.

In: Pictorial Essays … ISBN: 978-1-53618-014-5
Editors: PH Sugarbaker and RN Low ©2020 Nova Science Publishers, Inc.

Chapter 6

PERITONEAL METASTASES: THEIR ASSOCIATED CLINICAL FEATURES

Clarisse Dromain
University Hospital CHUV, Lausanne, Switzerland

INTRODUCTION

Imaging to detect peritoneal metastases remains a difficult task. Usually, the lesions are of small size. Consider also the peritoneal cavity's vast field for radiologic exploration and very obscure locations of some lesions. The knowledge of indirect signs of peritoneal metastases as well as mimickers can help to improve diagnostic accuracy and patient management. The associated clinical features inside and outside the peritoneal space can assist the radiologist in his/her best efforts.

ASCITES

First, is ascites a result of peritoneal metastases or caused by an unrelated condition? Ascites from peritoneal metastases is due to altered vascular permeability and obstructive lymphatic drainage. Malignant ascites account for only 7-10% of all cases of ascites [1]. So if your patient has ascites, in most of cases it would be due to a benign condition such as cirrhosis, congestive heart failure, nephrosis, pancreatitis, or peritonitis. Ascites is also present in cases of peritoneal metastases, more in some diagnoses than others. For example, we know that ascites is more often associated with ovarian cancer and peritoneal mesothelioma than for colorectal cancer. The presence of ascites in patients with known cancer indicates the need for a careful analysis of the peritoneal cavity to look for all the signs of peritoneal metastases. But the presence of ascites alone does not allow one to make the diagnosis of peritoneal metastases.

Table 6.1. Causes of ascites in patients with malignancy (From Reference [2])

Cause	Frequency among patients with malignancy-related ascites
Peritoneal metastases	53 percent
Massive liver metastases causing portal hypertension	13 percent
Peritoneal metastases plus massive liver metastases	13 percent
Hepatocellular carcinoma plus cirrhosis	13 percent
Chylous ascites due to malignancy, usually lymphoma	7 percent
Budd-Chiari syndrome due to malignancy occluding the hepatic veins	Rare

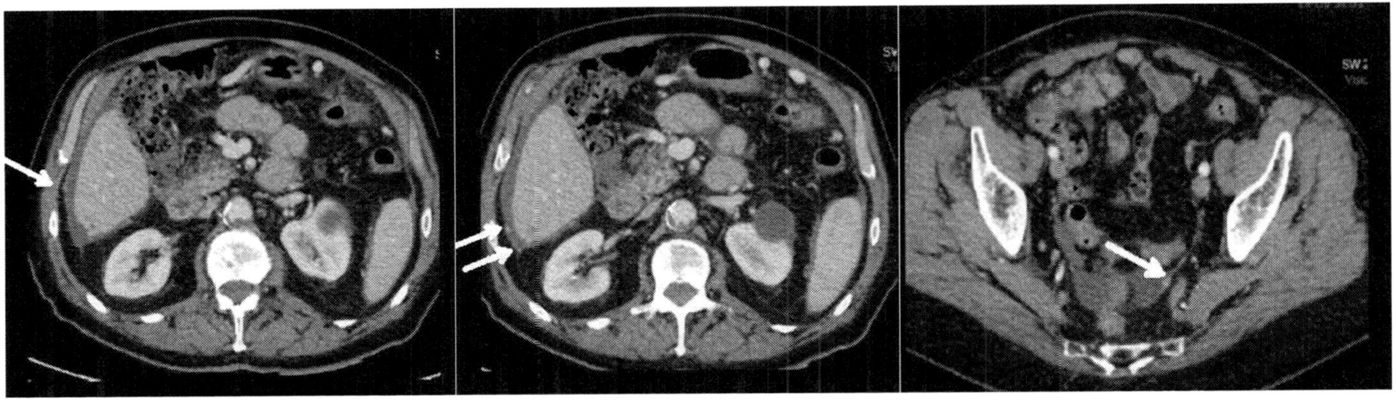

Figure 6.1. CT of the abdomen and pelvis in a patient with ascites. Small tumor implants are depicted beneath the right hemidiaphragm and in the pelvis.

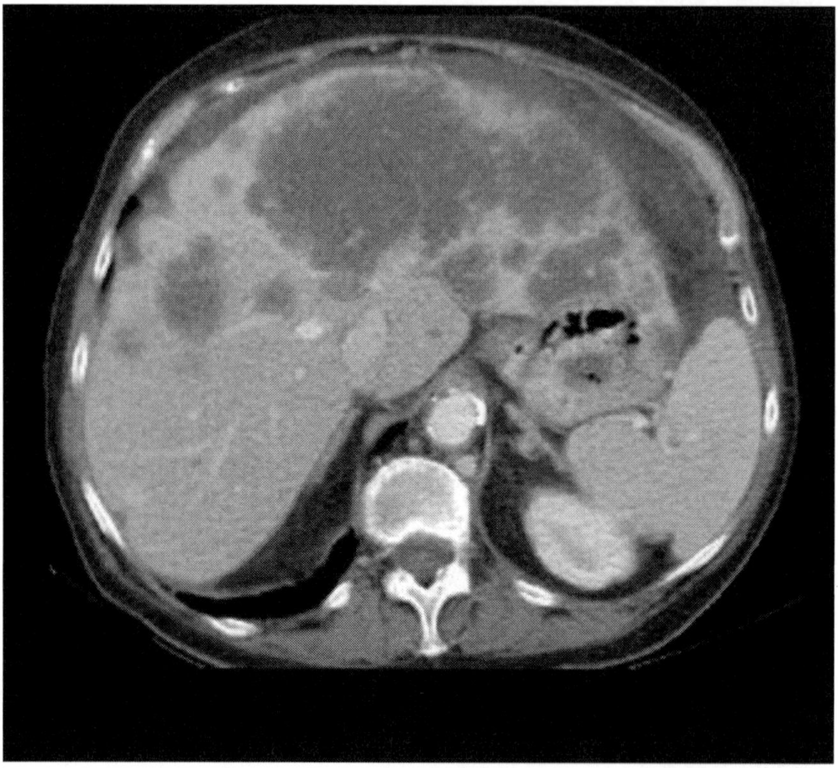

Figure 6.2. CT shows massive liver deposits from colon cancer with reactive ascites.

However, when ascites is present in a patient with peritoneal metastases we know that we are better able to depict small implants of tumor (Figure 6.1). We are able to see very small tumor implants on the parietal peritoneum. In the pelvis without ascites, probably we will not be able to see the small nodule at all. So in this case ascites was of help.

Table 6.1 shows that malignant disease can cause ascites by at least 6 different mechanisms [2]. Peritoneal metastases is one of them but you could have massive liver deposits causing portal hypertension. Figure 6.2 shows extensive liver metastases from colon cancer with reactive ascites but no peritoneal metastases. You could have ascites from hepatocellular carcinomatosis plus cirrhosis, chylous ascites due to malignancy, or Budd-Chiari syndrome due to malignant occlusion of the hepatic veins.

October 2015

July 2016

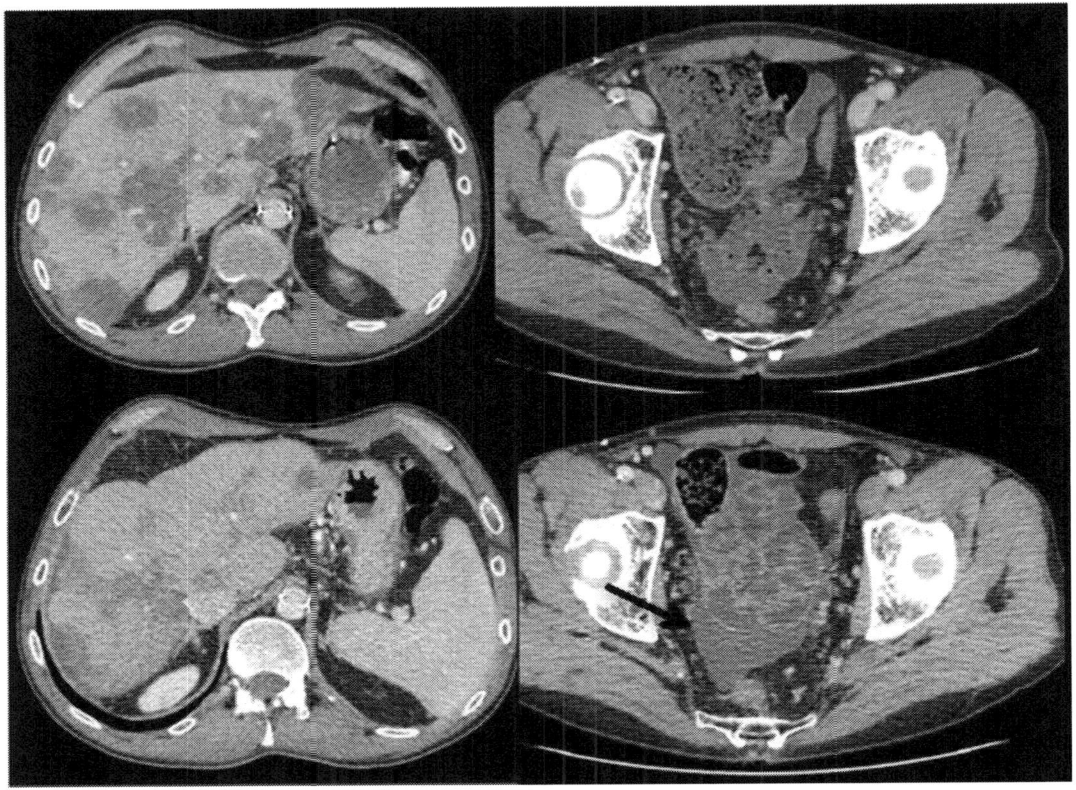

Figure 6.3. CT cuts of abdomen and pelvis in a patient treated with FOLFOX chemotherapy. Between October 2015 and July 2016 the liver metastases regressed. A syndrome of occlusive sinusoids resulted in the progression of ascites within the pelvis.

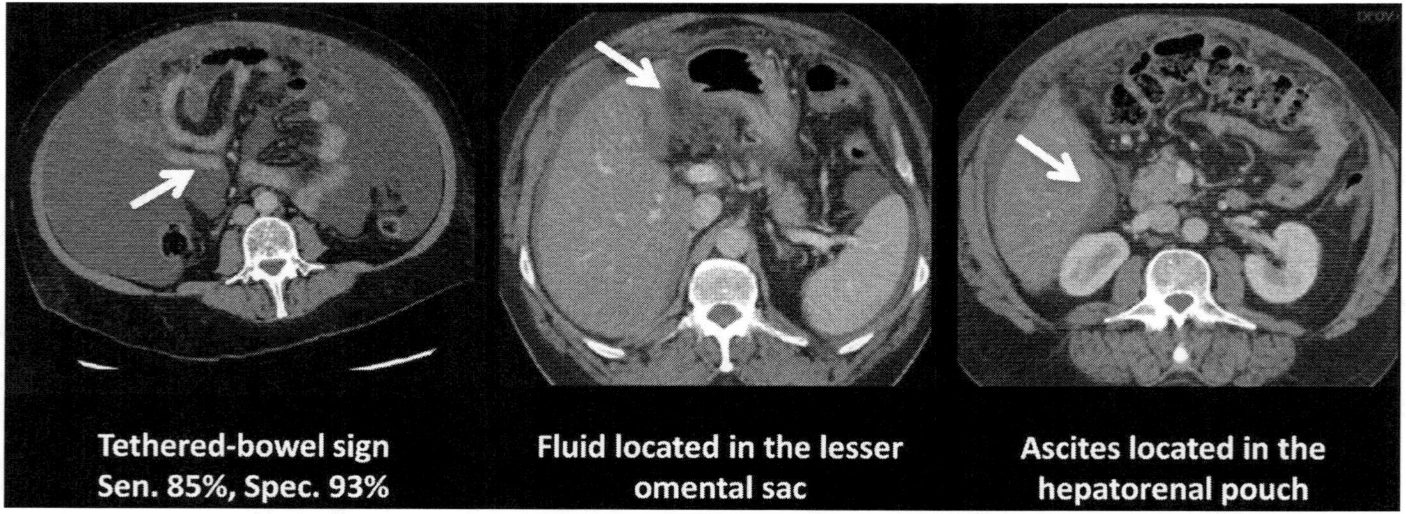

Figure 6.4. CT scan in a patient with peritoneal metastases layered out on the small bowel mesentery. Ascites in these patients often accumulates in the lesser omental sac and in the hepatorenal pouch.

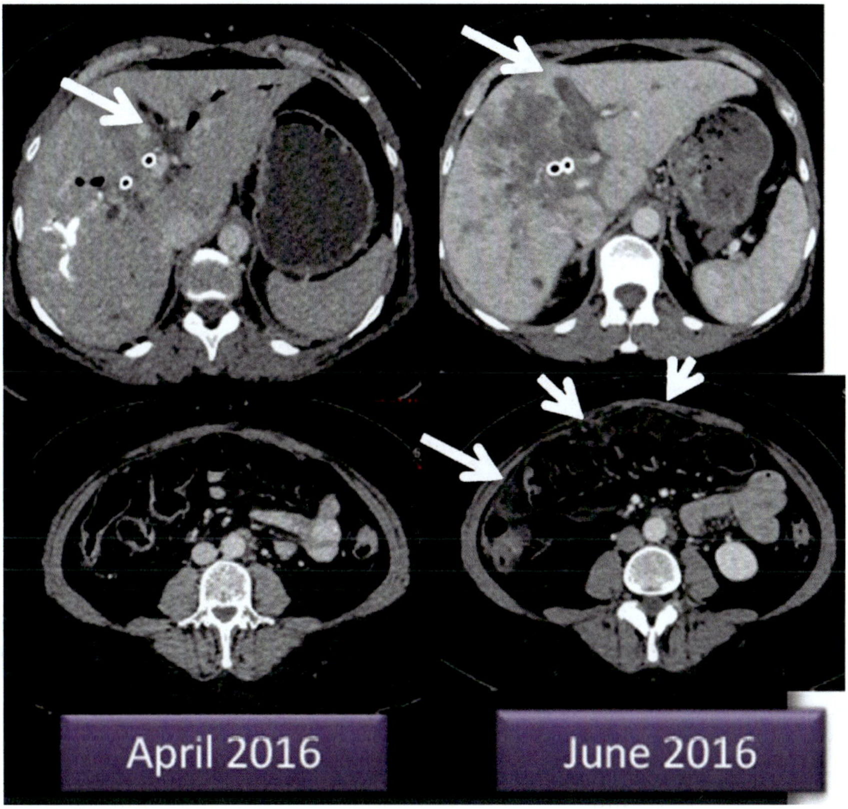

Figure 6.5. CT of the liver in a patient with involvement of the falciform ligament with rapid progression.

Figure 6.3 illustrates an interesting and possibly confusing case. This patient with colon cancer and liver metastases was treated with FOLFOX plus bevacizumab. You can see the very good response from October 2015 to July 2016 on liver metastases with fibrotic reaction. What did not correlate with a response was the appearance of fluid in the pelvis. The CEA tumor marker showed a substantial decrease. Again, a discordance between the appearance of fluid, the good response of liver metastases, and the very good response of marker. The answer is in the splenomegaly. We have an increase of the spleen so the diagnosis very suggestive of sinusoidal obstructive syndrome (SOS), due to chemotherapy particularly oxaliplatin [3].

As shown in Figure 6.4, ascites is commonly associated with peritoneal metastases layered out on the small bowel mesentery. There is a very high specific association of tethered bowel sign and fluid located in the lesser omental sac or ascites located in the hepatorenal pouch. Ascites in these locations is more likely due malignant tumor than a benign cause [4].

Visceral Peritoneal Metastases

Peritoneal metastases to visceral peritoneum may be obscure and often remains a challenge to appreciate. Infiltration of the Falciform ligament may be obvious but missed by many radiologists. You can see this in Figure 6.5. On April 2016, we have an involvement of the Falciform ligament. In June 2016, you can see that the patient progressed and there is now a huge increase of the infiltration of the hepatic lesion. Also now there is infiltration of the fat of the greater omentum. We must always look for infiltration of the Falciform ligament. It is often a very early finding and indicates the beginning of peritoneal dissemination.

Another manifestation of visceral peritoneal involvement is a segment of small bowel fixed to the parietal peritoneum and the appearance of blockage of free circulation of ascites. With this finding, you don't even have a nodule or thickening well depicted. You should suspect in follow-up peritoneal metastases from colon cancer. In these cases, preoperative PET-CT or MRI diffusion-weighted images could help to detect additional findings and be more confident to say "yes, this is a peritoneal metastases".

Another indirect sign is ureteral dilatation. Appearance of a dilated ureter in a patient in follow-up for digestive or ovarian cancer is highly suggestive of peritoneal metastases in the absence of an obvious stone. On CT it is very easy to detect ureteral stenosis and in most cases the tumor implant causing obstruction is not visualized. The PET-CT is often of help because we are sometimes able to see tracer uptake in the area of the obstruction. That indicates peritoneal metastases. In patients with ureteral dilatation, it is more often due to peritoneal metastases than lymph node involvement.

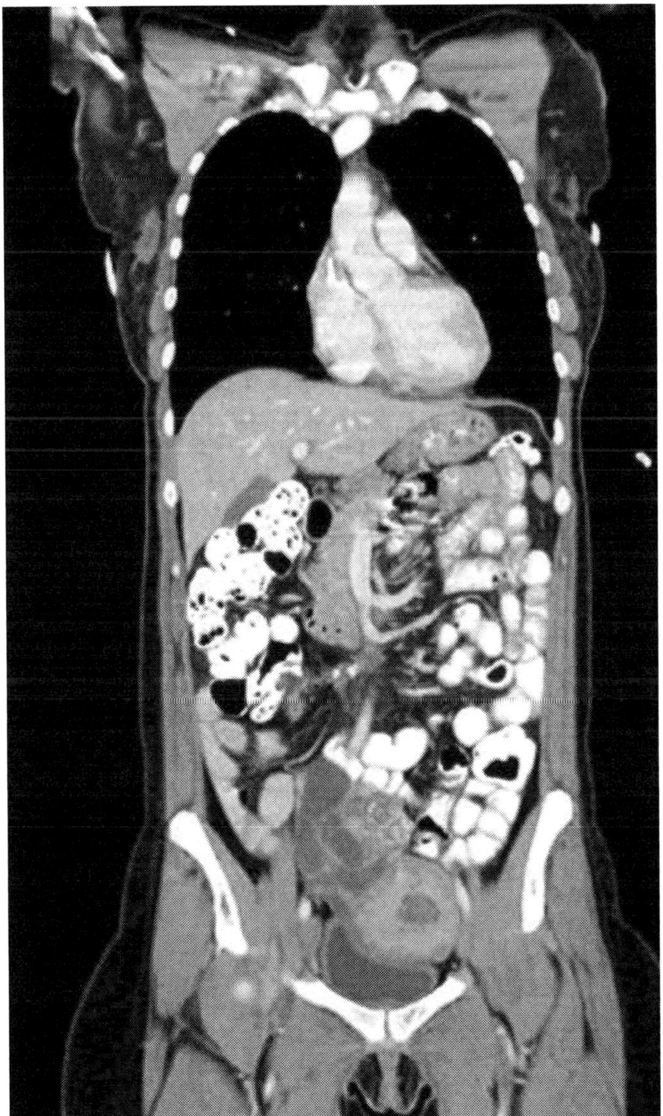

Figure 6.6. CT scan in a patient with right colon cancer and a synchronous large multicystic and solid right ovarian mass which is attached to the uterus. The primary lesion responded well to systemic chemotherapy but the ovarian metastasis progressed.

Colorectal cancer is the most common non-gynecologic malignancy causing ovarian metastases with a rate of 1-10% for synchronous cancer and 1-2% for metachronous disease. The ovarian masses are often voluminous, cystic, mucinous and symptomatic (Figure 6.6). A very important point is that ovarian metastases are less responsive to systemic chemotherapy than the other site of disease. That means that you should not choose this ovarian metastases as an indicator lesion if you want to assess, for example, chemotherapy. Secondly, surgical resection of ovarian metastases should be discussed, even in the palliative setting. We know that gastrointestinal surgeons prefer not to perform palliative surgery. But in this case one must perform a debulking to remove the ovarian metastases and then give conventional chemotherapy for palliative treatment. We know also that ovarian metastases are frequently associated with additional peritoneal metastases. In the study by Goere et al., when peritoneal metastases of a primary colorectal or appendiceal cancer are confirmed, at least 52% of ovaries will have synchronous metastases [5]. Therefore, the presence of ovarian masses, in particular, large cystic masses on CT images in colorectal cancer should prompt careful analysis of the peritoneal cavity. It is really a very suggestive sign of peritoneal disease and may be an indication to perform reoperative surgery [6].

Another associated clinical and radiologic feature is the Sister Mary Joseph nodule, a malignant metastatic umbilical nodule (Figure 6.7). The proposed route for the spread of cancer to the umbilicus includes direct extension from the peritoneum or spread via arterial, venous, and lymphatic channels. It is most commonly found in association with adenocarcinoma but not with other types of cancer and the most common primary site includes the stomach, ovary, colon, and pancreas.

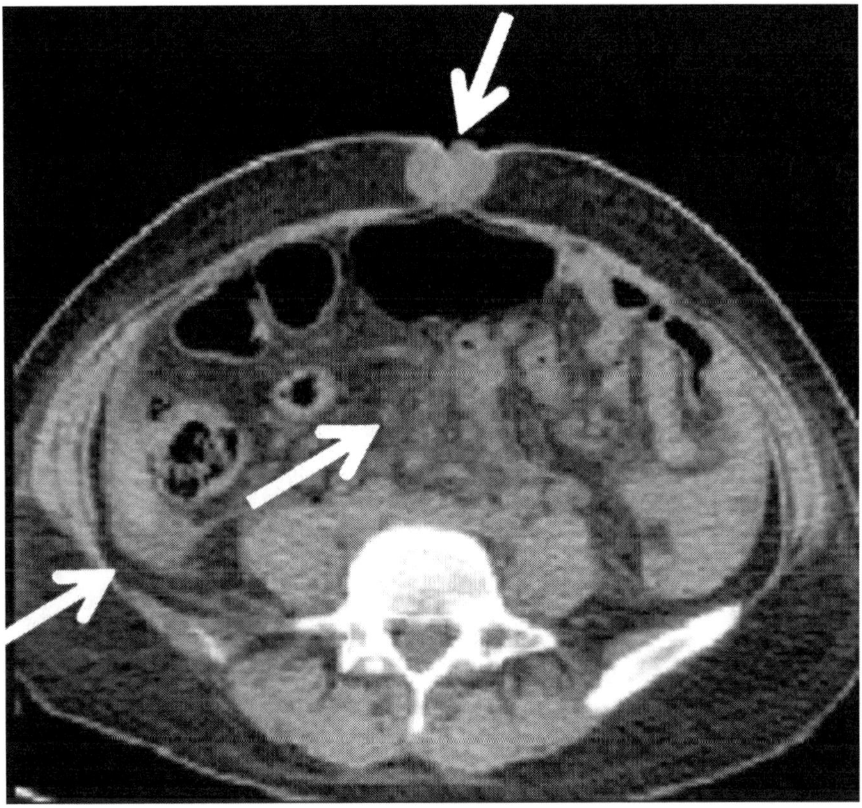

Figure 6.7. The CT shows a malignant metastatic nodule within the umbilicus. Also shown by the arrows are ascites in the right paracolic sulcus and nodularity of the mesentery.

IMAGING THE CARDIOPHRENIC ANGLE LYMPH NODE

Other imaging feature is cardiophrenic angle lymph node (CPALN). These are the lymph nodes located in an area adjacent to the pericardium within 2 cm of the diaphragm. In fact, the CPALN chain is a major lymph drainage system of both the peritoneum and the diaphragm muscle. So you could have CPALN involvement if you have disease of the peritoneum or disease of the diaphragm. In fact, for the peritoneal lymphatic pathway there are two different pathways.

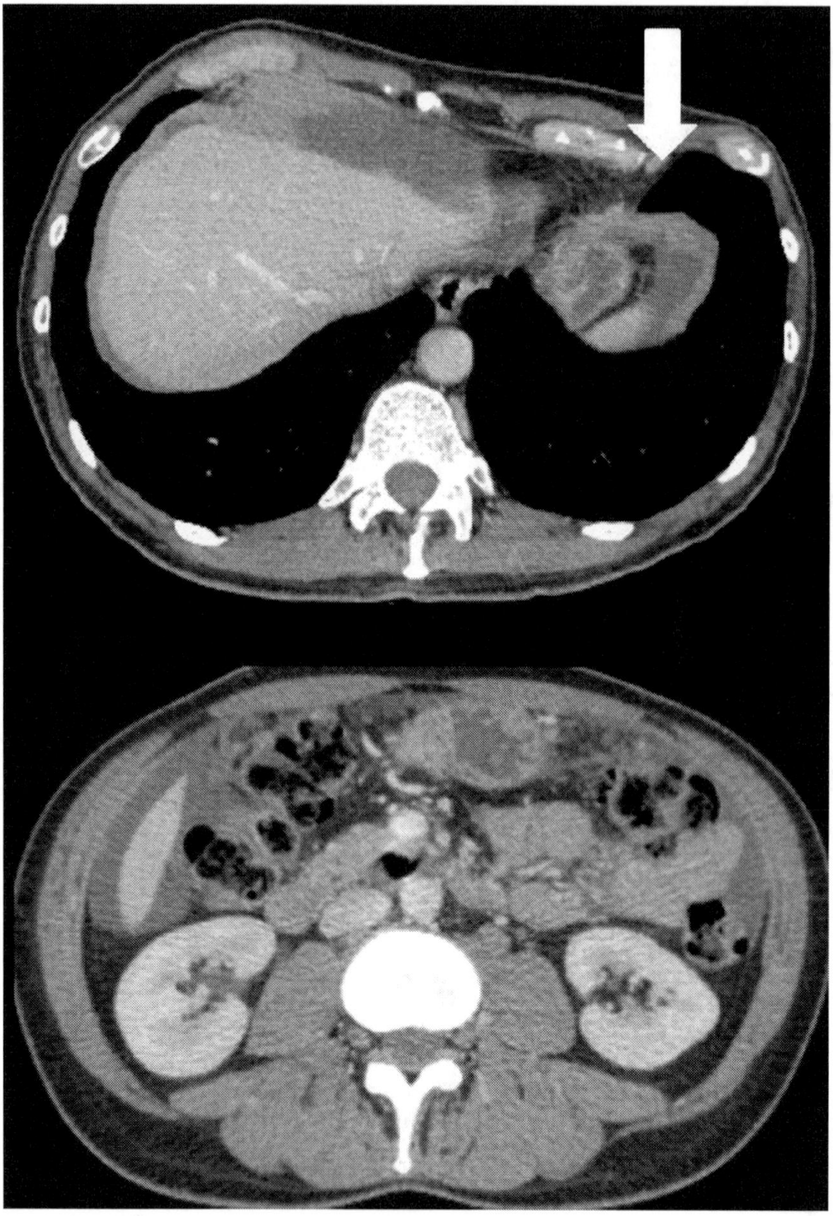

Figure 6.8. CT in an ovarian cancer patient that shows a cardiophrenic angle lymph node (CPALN). In this patient a cut through mid-abdomen shows ascites in the right and left paracolic sulcus and nodularity of the greater omentum. CPALN is an indicator of advanced disease.

The first is lymphatic vessels of the diaphragm that are arranged as two plexi, one on the peritoneal surface and one on the pleura surface that intercommunicate. Then these plexi go into collecting ducts associated with the internal mammary vessels. This means that lymph is collected at the anterior part of the thorax along the sternum and then goes to the anterior mediastinal lymph nodes in the region of the thymus. The second pathway is the more common pathway coming from the celiac, superior mesenteric, and periportal lymph node to the mediastinal lymph node and finally to the thoracic duct.

The CPALN has been described in ovarian cancer and associated with very advanced peritoneal metastases. In the study by Hynninen, 30 women with advanced ovarian cancer were evaluated [7]. They did PET-CT in all cases. They depicted cardiophrenic lymph node in 67% of patients by PET whereas only 33% were depicted using CT. Patients that have cardiophrenic lymph node had significantly more ascites, higher CA-125 tumor marker level, and more frequent peritoneal metastases compared to patients without CPALN. Figure 6.8 shows a very small CPALN on the left side associated with peritoneal metastases.

We did a study in 550 patients with colorectal cancer treated by surgery with complete peritoneal exploration. We found the presence of the CPALN in 45% of CT images [8]. These ranged from 1-6 lymph nodes per patient with a median size of 7 mm. In the top of Table 6.2, concerning all patients, you see a selection bias because we have a lot of peritoneal metastases patients in our population. Thirty percent of our patients with colorectal cancer had PM because we are a dedicated center for HIPEC. So you see that the sensitivity for the detection of peritoneal metastases due to the presence of CPALN was 75% with a very high negative predictive value of 86%. In the bottom portion of Table 6.2, we consider patients with no obvious sign of PM on CT and only CPALN. The sensitivity was lower but the negative predictive value was very high at 91%. It means that if you don't have the CPALN on a normal CT, the probability to have peritoneal metastases is very low. And the opposite is true. If you have CPALN, you should carefully analyze the peritoneum to look for the presence of peritoneal carcinomatosis.

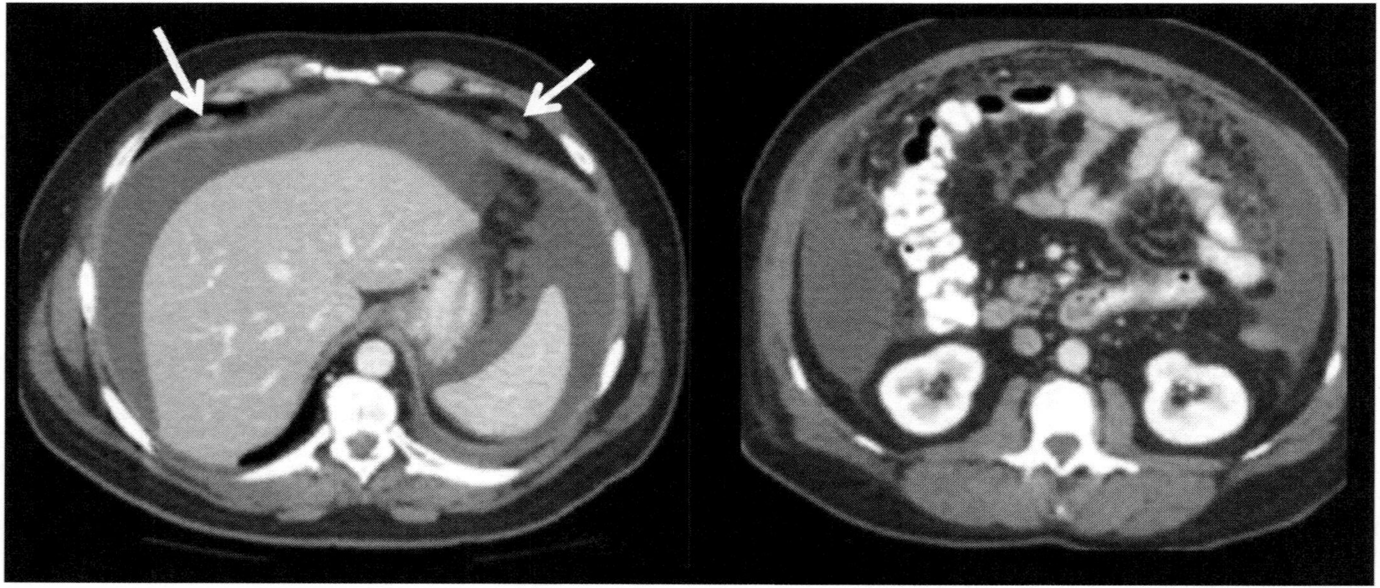

Figure 6.9. Cardiophrenic angle lymph nodes in an ovarian cancer patient with ascites and omental and mesenteric disease.

Table 6.2. Cardiophrenic angle lymph nodes (CPALN) in 550 patients with colorectal cancer

ALL PATIENTS (n = 550)			
	PM (n = 165) 30%		**No PM (n = 385)**
CPALN (%)			
Yes	123 (75%)		122 (32%)
No	42 (25%)		263 (68%)
Sens	**Spec**	**PPV**	**NPV**
75%	68%	50%	86%
Patients with No Obvious PM on CT (n = 451)			
	CP (n = 66)		**No CP (n = 385)**
CPALN (%)			
Yes	41 (62%)		120 (31%)
No	25 (38%)		265 (69%)
Sens	**Spec**	**PPV**	**NPV**
62%	69%	25%	91%

(PM = peritoneal metastases, Sens = sensitivity, Spec = specificity, PPV = positive predictive value, NPV = negative predictive value, from Reference [9] with permission)

Figure 6.9 is an example of a patient with CPALN, ascites, huge involvement of the greater omentum, and the mesentery. This patient had cytoreductive surgery and then HIPEC. The CPALN were involved by cancer

Using the same group of patients, we did a retrospective analysis to assess the prognostic impact of the presence of CPALN [9]. We analyzed 114 patients with peritoneal metastases from colorectal cancer treated with cytoreductive surgery and HIPEC (Table 6.3). The mean PCI score was 9 and 21% of patients had associated liver metastases; 71% of the women had ovarian metastases. The median follow-up was 4 years and the presence of visible CPALN in patients was 64%. We did not find an impact on overall survival nor on progression-free survival, unlike the PCI score. In patients treated with cytoreductive surgery and HIPEC we did not find a prognostic impact of the presence of CPALN.

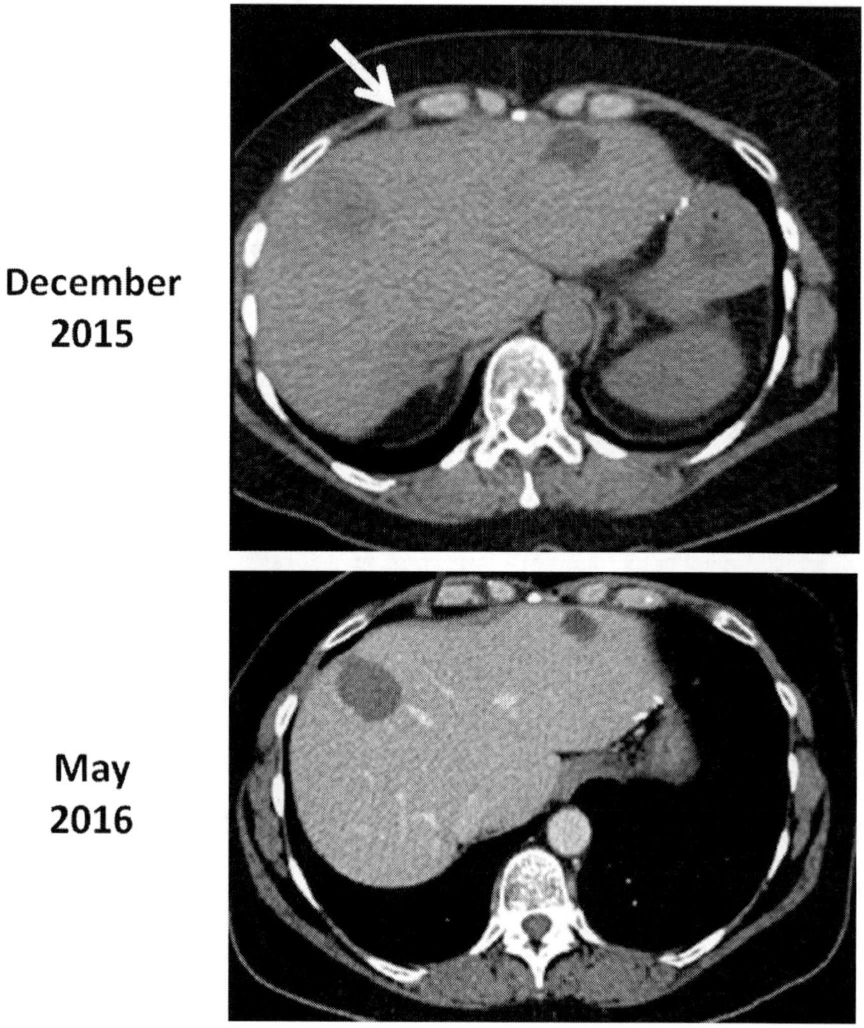

Figure 6.10. CT of a patient with gastric cancer, CPALN metastasis, and liver metastasis. On FOLFOX chemotherapy both the liver metastasis and the CPALN metastasis decreased in size.

In a more recent study by Jeune et al., they assessed 91 patients undergoing colectomy for colon cancer [10]. They had an incidence of CPALN of about 40% in this non-selected series of patients. The number of patients with peritoneal metastases was much lower than in our study, only 6%. So the clinical features associated with the presence of CPALN on multivariate analysis were distant metastases and the absence of mucinous adenocarcinoma. Patients with CPALN had similar overall survival but decreased progression-free survival. However, there was no significant correlation on the multivariate analysis. So the conclusion of these authors was that the CPALN is mainly an indicator of metastatic spread of colorectal cancer regardless of the location of the metastases. In the absence of CPALN, peritoneal metastases can almost be excluded because of a very high negative predictive value.

Table 6.3. Prognostic impact of cardiophrenic angle lymph nodes (CPALN) in 114 patients with peritoneal metastases from colorectal cancer (CRC) treated with cytoreductive surgery (CRS) and HIPEC

- 114 patients with PM from CRC treated with CRS + HIPEC
  - Mean PCI score = 9.2
  - 21% had associated liver metastases
  - 71% of the women had ovarian metastases
- Median follow-up 3.9 years
- Presence of CPALN in 64% of patients
- CPALN had no impact on OS nor DFS, unlike the PCI score

(PCI = peritoneal cancer index, OS = overall survival, DFS = disease-free survival, from Reference [8] with permission)

Another important question, is the CPALN malignant? The primary surgeon is reluctant to remove it as part of a surgical procedure because it is above the diaphragm. In the study from Yoo et al., 11 patients with ovarian carcinoma and peritoneal metastases had cytoreductive surgery and systematic dissection of the CPALN [11]. When the node was greater than 5 mm they did a transabdominal dissection through incised or resected diaphragm and the additional operation time was about 30 minutes. They found that the CPALN was involved by the tumor in 45% of patients. It is my opinion that it is really important to clearly state in our radiology report the presence of CPALN. The surgeon should consider removing it to have a complete resection in patients with peritoneal metastases.

Figure 6.10 shows a gastric adenocarcinoma treated with FOLFOX. There were peritoneal metastases and also liver metastases. Under treatment there was a good response of the liver metastases. There is also a decrease of the size of the CPALN suggestive that this lymph node was malignant.

Figure 6.11 shows a patient with a neuroendocrine tumor. On MRI, there is a CPALN with a very high enhancement suggestive of hypervascularity and malignant infiltration. Also, on F-DOPA PET there is high tracer uptake confirming that this lymph node was malignant.

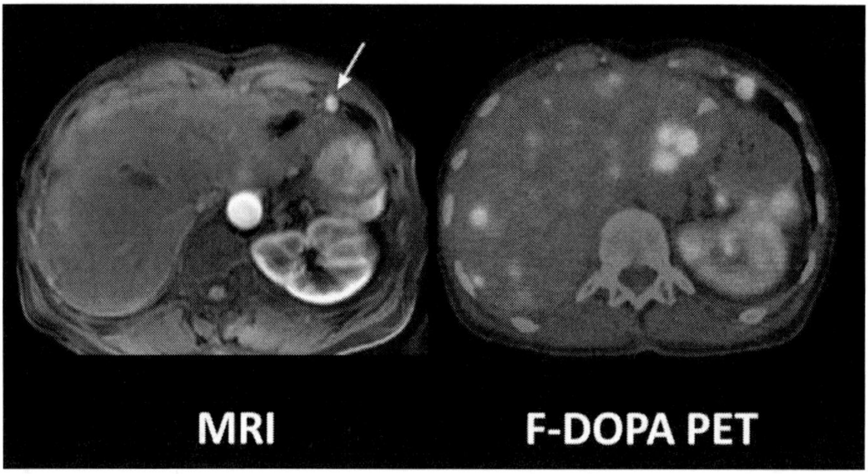

Figure 6.11. A neuroendocrine tumor which shows a cardiophrenic angle lymph node by MRI and by F-DOPA PET.

In summary, questions still exist but it is safe to say that CPALN increases the possibility of metastatic spread in ovarian and colorectal cancer. If CPALN are present, peritoneal metastases must be suspected in patients without obvious metastatic disease on preoperative imaging work-up. If there are isolated CPALN do additional investigations such as PET-CT, MRI, laparoscopy, or just careful postoperative follow-up. We don't have enough data to recommend a precise treatment plan for CPALN and a systematic node dissection is still under debate.

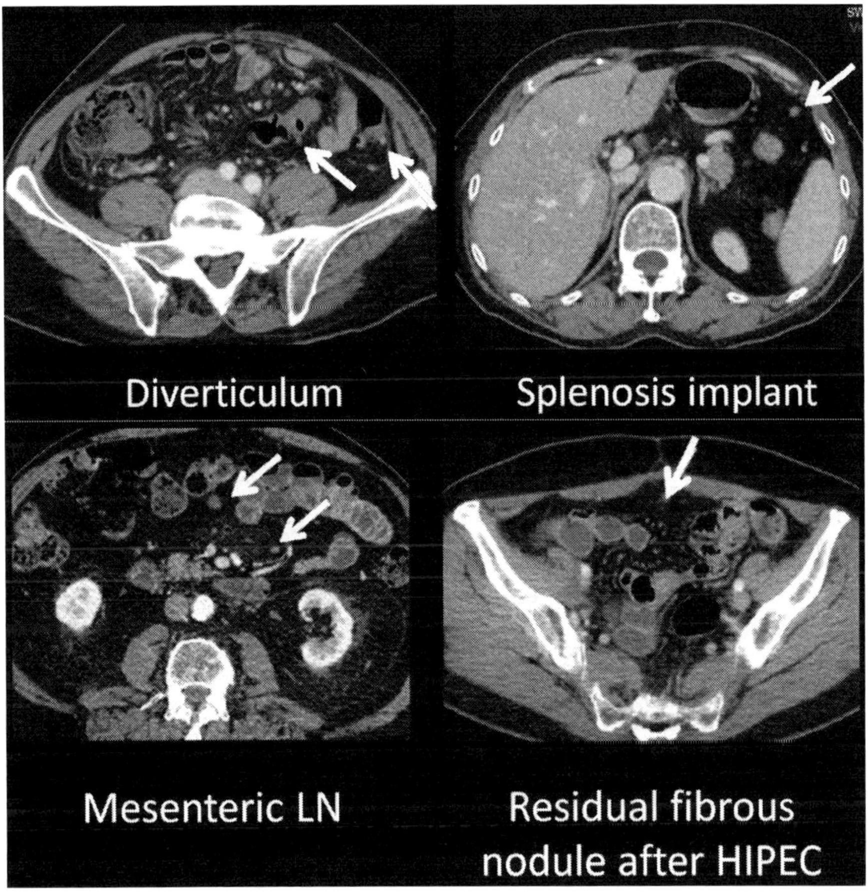

Figure 6.12. Peritoneal metastases mimickers by CT include a sigmoid colon diverticulum, splenosis implant, prominent mesenteric lymph node, and a postoperative fibrous nodule.

PERITONEAL METASTASES MIMICKERS

There are a number of benign conditions that can be misinterpreted for peritoneal metastases. Figure 6.12. shows a sigmoid colon diverticulum, splenosis implant, prominent mesenteric lymph nodes, and a postoperative fibrous nodule. A colonic diverticulum may be easy to differentiate from tumor implant because it may show air filling. Mesenteric lymph nodes are tricky but most of the lymph nodes are close to the vessels and oval-shaped as compared to peritoneal implants which closer to the serosa of the bowel. More confusing, after cytoreduction and HIPEC are many postoperative changes. It is important to have a baseline postoperative CT about 2 months after surgery to be able to depict postoperative changes and then to follow the patient. This avoids false positive interpretations. Sometimes we encounter the same with perihepatic scalloping because surgeons do a lot of peritonectomy during the HIPEC procedure and you could misinterpret this as residual tumor. So always ask for a baseline postoperative follow-up CT.

Figure 6.13 shows a patient, 55 years old who had surgery for colon cancer 2 years prior. On the CT follow-up we find this peritoneal nodule also highly intense on PET. You can clearly see the nodule on the coronal reconstruction. In this patient, to make a diagnosis a reoperative surgery was performed. It was a desmoid tumor related to the prior surgical intervention.

Figure 6.14 shows a 55-year-old male with obstructing sigmoid colon cancer. We have some ascites fluid close to the descending colon. Be careful because when you have an obstructive colon cancer, you could have a benign peritoneal reaction. This patient was operated for the primary tumor. There was no peritoneal metastases but just inflammation. So be very careful in cases of obstruction. Don't go directly to the diagnosis of peritoneal metastases because this may cause the patient to be treated palliatively. He should be operated.

In summary, visualization of indirect signs of peritoneal metastases such as ovarian metastases, CPALN, fixation and agglutination of small bowel require a careful review of the peritoneal cavity and peritoneal folds. The interest of additional investigation should be discussed during multidisciplinary tumor board meetings including MRI, PET-CT, laparoscopy, or close follow-up. Further studies are mandatory to better understand the prognostic significance of CPALN and the need, or not, to perform their surgical removal.

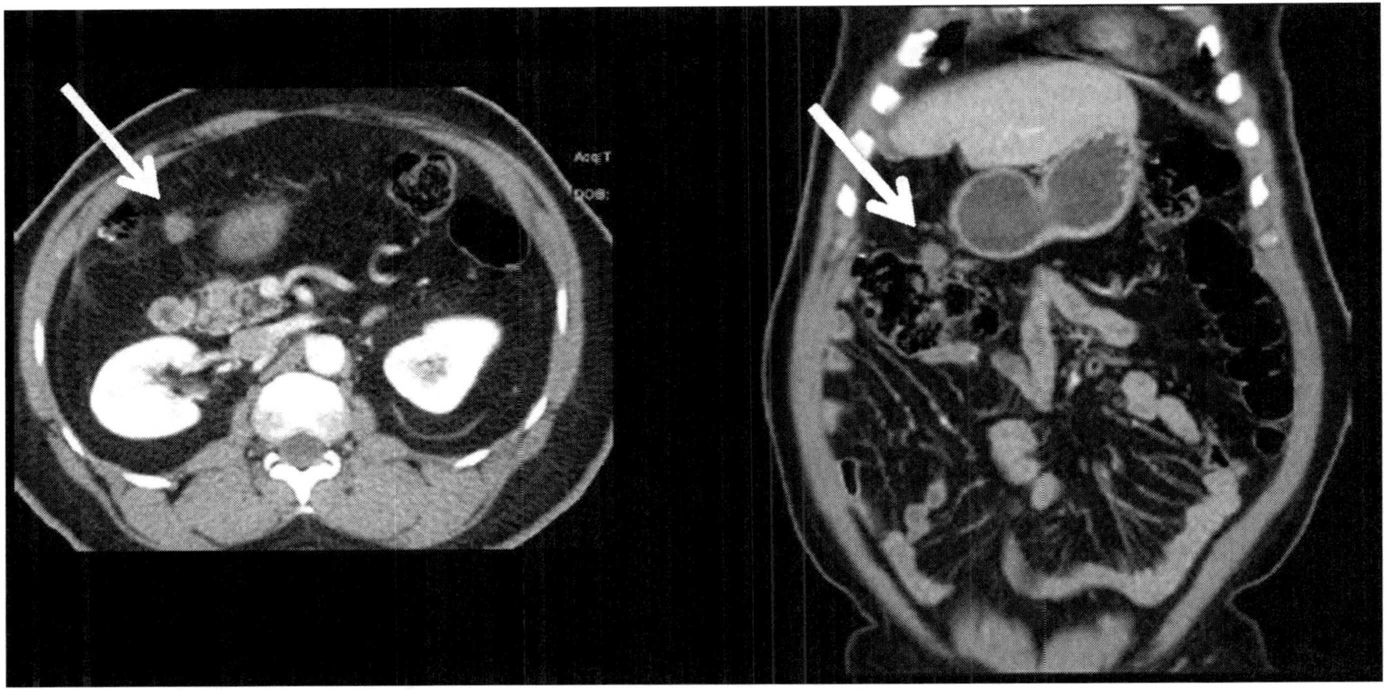

Figure 6.13. CT performed in follow-up shows a peritoneal nodule that was also highly intense on PET. Reoperative surgery was performed and shown to be a desmoid tumor.

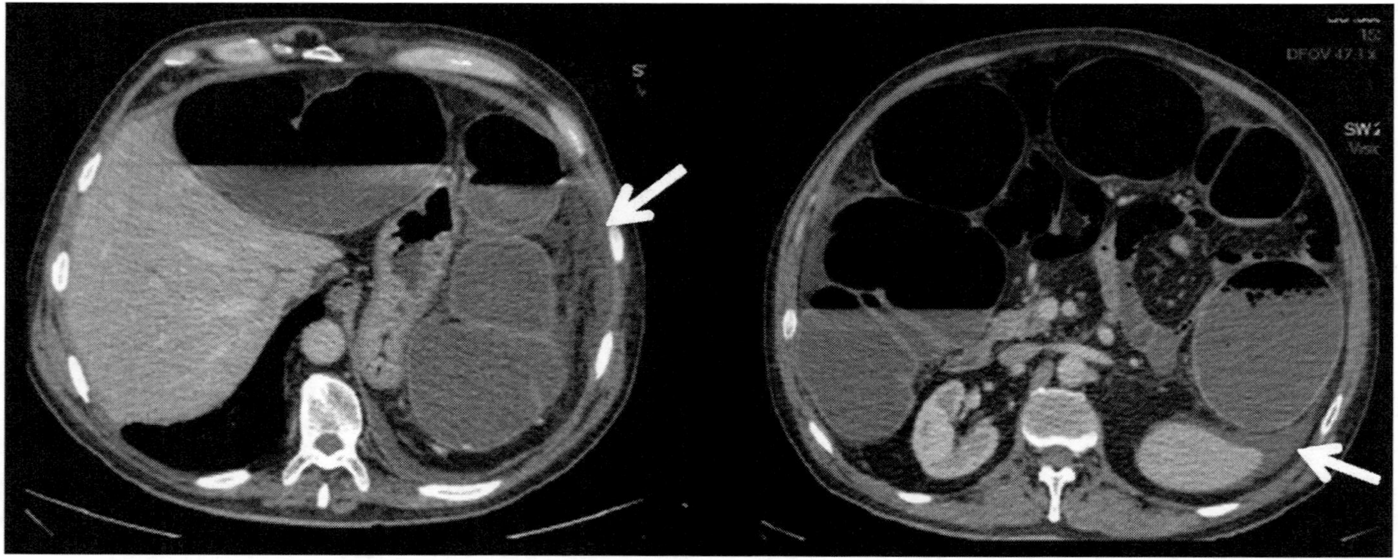

Figure 6.14. CT of an obstructing sigmoid colon cancer which shows ascites fluid. At surgery there was inflammation but no peritoneal metastases.

References

[1] Sangisetty, SL; Miner, TJ. Malignant ascites: A review of prognostic factors, pathophysiology and therapeutic measures. *World J Gastrointest Surg*, 2012, 4(4), 87-95.

[2] Runyon, BA; Hoefs, JC; Morgan, TR. Ascitic fluid analysis in malignancy-related ascites. *Hepatology*, 1988, 8, 1104-1109.

[3] Valla, DC; Cazals-Hatem, D. Sinusoidal obstruction syndrome. *Clin Res Hepatol Gastroenterol*, 2016, 40(4), 378-385.

[4] Seltzer, SE. Analysis of the tethered-bowel sign on abdominal CT as a predictor of malignant ascites. *Gastrointest Radiol*, 1987, 12, 245-249.

[5] Goere, D; Daveau, C; Elias, D; et al. The differential response to chemotherapy of ovarian metastases from colorectal carcinoma. *Eur J Surg Oncol*, 2008, 34(12), 1335-1339.

[6] Elias, D; Goere, D; Di Pietrantonio, D; et al. Results of systematic second-look surgery in patients at high risk of developing colorectal peritoneal carcinomatosis. *Ann Surg*, 2008, 247, 445-450.

[7] Hynninen, J; Auranen, A; Carpén, O; et al. FDG PET/CT in staging of advanced epithelial ovarian cancer: frequency of supradiaphragmatic lymph node metastasis challenges the traditional pattern of disease spread. *Gynecol Oncol*, 2012, 126(1), 64-68.

[8] Caramella, C; Pottier, E; Borget, I; et al. Value of cardiophrenic angle lymph node for the diagnosis of colorectal peritoneal carcinomatosis. *Eur J Cancer*, 2013, 49(18), 3798-3805.

[9] Elias, D; Borget, I; Farron, M; et al. Prognostic significance of visible cardiophrenic angle lymph nodes in the presence of peritoneal metastases from colorectal cancers. *Eur J Surg Oncol*, 2013, 39(11), 1214-1218.

[10] Jeune, F; Brouquet, A; Caramella, C; et al. Cardiophrenic angle lymph node is an indicator of metastatic spread but not specifically peritoneal carcinomatosis in colorectal cancer patients: Results of a prospective validation study in 91 patients. *Eur J Surg Oncol*, 2016, 42(6), 861-868.

[11] Yoo, HJ; Lim, MC; Song, YJ; Jung, YS; Kim, SH; Yoo, CW; Park, SY. Transabdominal cardiophrenic lymph node dissection (CPLND) via incised diaphragm replace conventional video-assisted thoracic surgery for cytoreductive surgery in advanced ovarian cancer. *Gynecol Oncol*, 2013, 129(2), 341-345.

In: Pictorial Essays …
ISBN: 978-1-53618-014-5
Editors: PH Sugarbaker and RN Low

Chapter 7

THE MINIMUM REQUIRED REPORT FOR PERITONEAL METASTASES

Pascal Rousset, MD, PhD
Department of Radiology,
Lyon Sud University Hospital, Lyon, France

INTRODUCTION

Currently, the responsibilities of the radiologist to provide a concise and accurate written report for a patient with peritoneal metastases are greater than ever due to increasing number of patients undergoing surgical intervention. An accurate imaging analysis of the extent and distribution of the peritoneal metastases assists in patient selection to avoid open and close surgery due to an unresectable lesion or high tumor volume. It also provides crucial information to the surgeon regarding the resections that will be required for complete cytoreductive surgery and thus optimizes the planning of resources preoperatively. Information from imaging will assist the surgeon in consenting the patient regarding the surgical procedure as extensive surgery is demanding and stressful for patients and adds significant morbidity. A minimal and standardized report is required to provide maximal useful information. The report can be divided into five steps: the first three steps describe peritoneal metastases, the fourth step evaluates extraperitoneal metastases and the final fifth step determines the location of the primary cancer in case of initial staging.

First Step: Establish the Presence versus Absence of Peritoneal Metastases

The first step is an attempt to establish the presence or absence of peritoneal metastases. The radiologist must have extensive expertise because it is often difficult to identify the peritoneal metastases. The radiologist should search through the images in a clockwise manner, the same as the peritoneal fluid circulation, to look at each abdominal and pelvic region. Signs of peritoneal metastases include the presence of nodules, peritoneal thickening, or areas of fat stranding. Detection of peritoneal metastases is, of course, important for patient management but also in clinical research because the presence of peritoneal metastases often excludes patients from clinical research projects.

The radiologist must also have extensive expertise to avoid false positive interpretations caused by mimickers of peritoneal metastases. Knowledge of the malignancy being imaged as well as the appearance of the different manifestations of known peritoneal disease helps the radiologist to see what may not be obvious. Also, the radiologist needs to avoid false positive interpretations due to postoperative changes. Baseline postoperative imaging is mandatory otherwise changes caused by prior surgical interventions will be very misleading (Figure 7.1). The radiologist has to report if these changes are stable, resolved, or progressing which is indicative for recurrence.

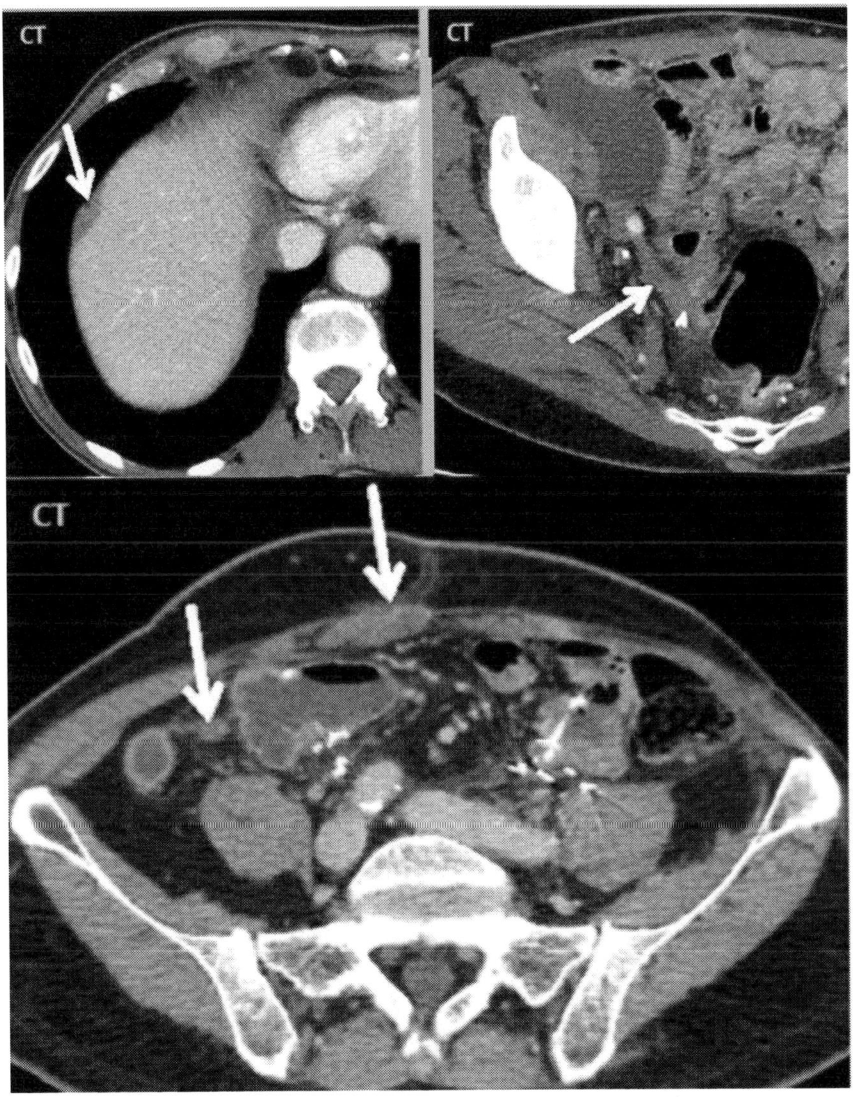

Figure 7.1. Postoperative changes (arrows) in the liver capsule, pelvic peritoneum, and abdominal incision which may be a trap of false positive findings.

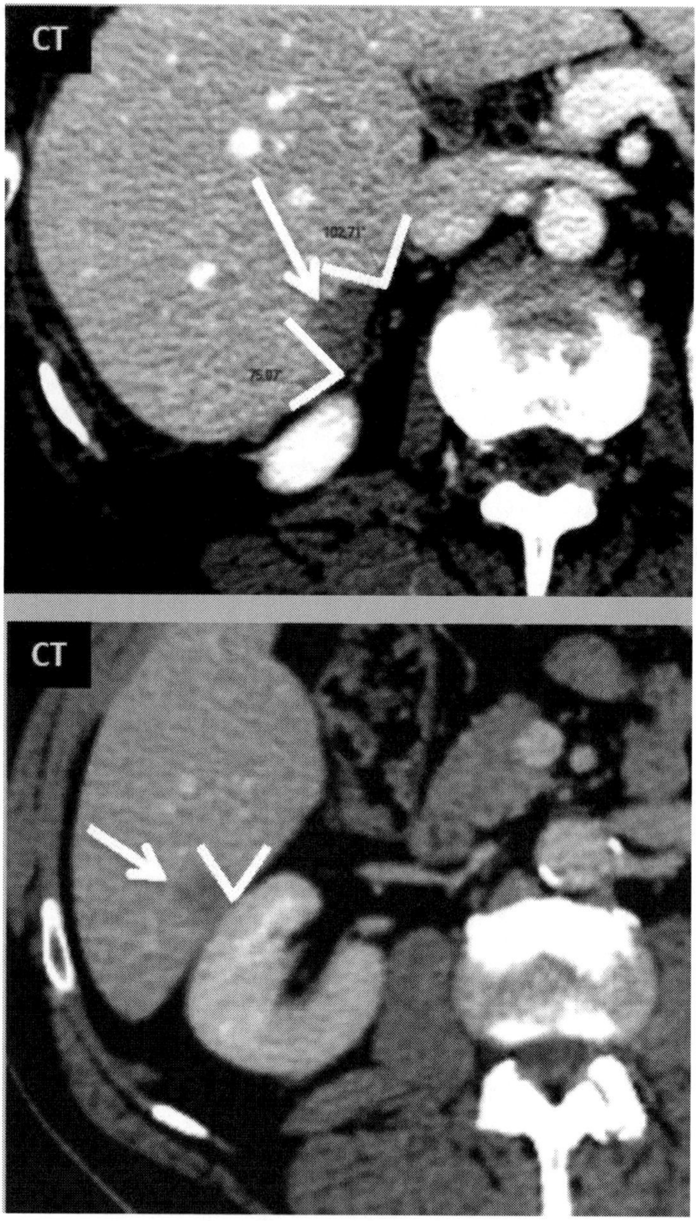

Figure 7.2. Top. The presence of at least one obtuse angle of the liver lesion of an ovarian cancer with the liver capsule (arrow) suggests a peritoneal metastases rather than an intraparenchymal blood borne metastases. Bottom. The acute angle of the liver lesion of a colorectal cancer with the liver capsule (arrow) suggests a hematogenous metastasis.

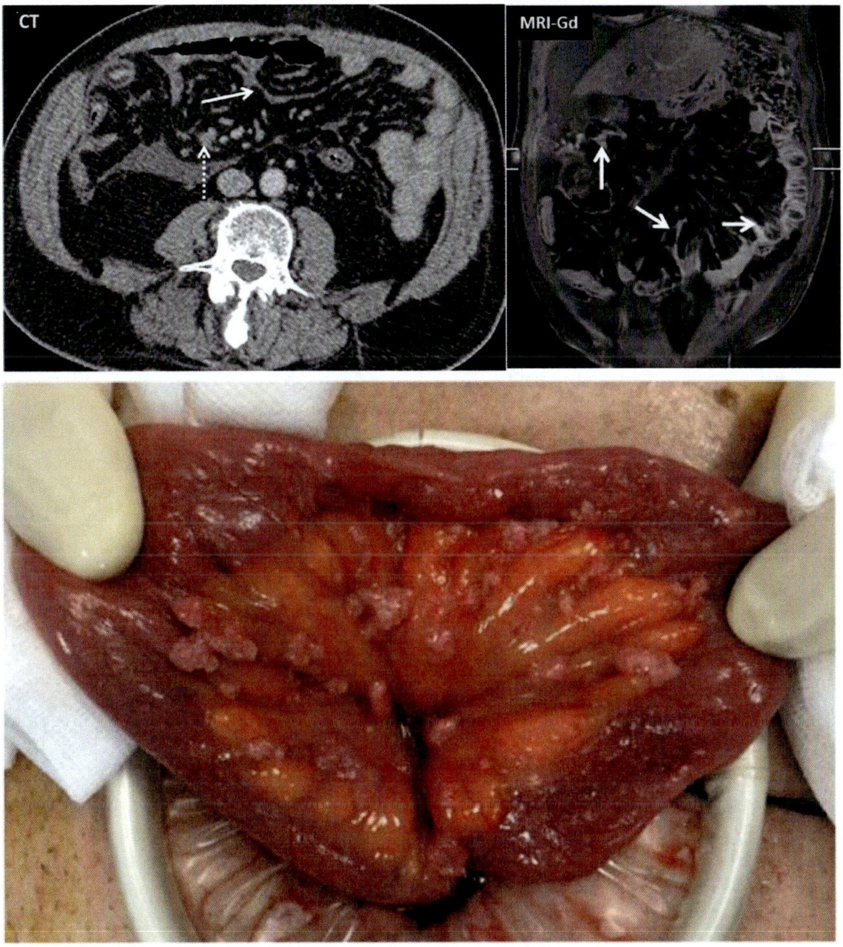

Figure 7.3. Top. The mesenteric nodules are between the vessels suggesting peritoneal implants rather than lymph nodes (dashed arrow), while vegetations from the mesentery suggest peritoneal metastases (arrow). Bottom. Intraoperative photograph showing papillary mesothelioma.

Oftentimes the radiologist has to decide if the nodules are intrinsic or extrinsic on the surface of the liver or on the spleen. The management of the patient will be different. The radiologist has to consider the shape, the form and angle between the lesion and the adjacent parenchyma. In Figure 7.2 top, the shape of the lesion is oval and the angle of the nodule with the liver surface is obtuse, suggesting the lesion is extrinsic with peritoneal metastases. In Figure 7.2 bottom, the liver lesion is more round with an acute angle and is likely a parenchymal liver metastasis. In doubtful cases, the radiologist should suggest another imaging technique. MRI may provide more confidence in concluding that a lesion is liver metastases rather than a peritoneal metastasis because of the signal and the peripheral enhancement.

Another difficult situation is to determine if nodules in the mesentery are mesenteric lymph nodes or peritoneal metastases. Schematically, lymph nodes are close to the vessels within the fat, mostly oval or round and well defined. In contrast, as seen in Figure 7.3 top left, peritoneal nodules are between vessels with a more or less sheet-like configuration on the bowel serosa. In Figure 7.3 top right, numerous vegetations are seen on the visceral peritoneum. It was a papillary mesothelioma (Figure 7.3 bottom).

Second Step: Qualitative Analysis of Peritoneal Metastases

When the diagnosis of peritoneal metastases has been established, the second step is to qualitatively describe three types of lesions.

Detection of Unresectable Lesions through Identification of Concerning Radiologic Features

The first type of lesion in the qualitative analysis are those that are likely to be unresectable lesions. The concept of unresectability is complex and difficult, mostly depending on patient age and status, the primary cancer (invasive versus non-invasive histopathology), and the tumor distribution and volume [1-5]. The presence of extensive lesions at particular anatomic sites may be absolutely non-resectable and preclude surgery and sometimes they are only suggestive of non-resectability [3].

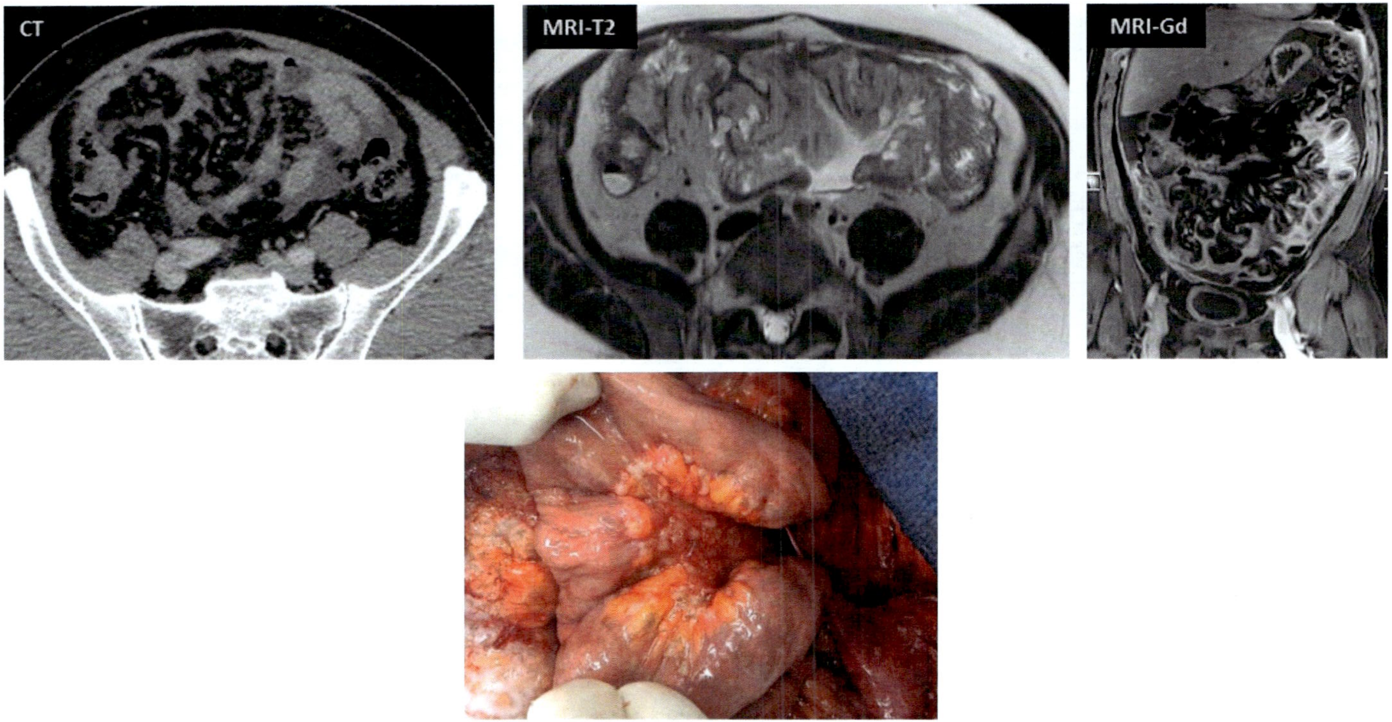

Figure 7.4. Top. A large volume of mucinous tumor that diffusely involves the small bowel mesentery. MRI was more accurate to depict the extent of disease than CT. Bottom. Intraoperative photograph of the extensive mucinous tumor on the mesentery.

The three more frequent sites for unresectable lesions are small bowel and its mesentery, the porta hepatis, and pelvis. Some other concerning radiologic features may not preclude surgery by themselves. A single concerning radiologic features will often add complexity to the cytoreductive surgery yet resection scored as complete, while two or more concerning radiologic features usually indicates a suboptimal resection [3-5]. These features are described in the next paragraph.

Regarding concerning radiologic features whose mere presence may preclude surgery, the radiologist must pay special attention to three anatomic sites.

Diffuse small bowel involvement is sometimes difficult to depict, but when present the radiologist has to estimate the extent of involvement as more or less than 50% of the bowel [6]. In the pseudomyxoma peritonei shown in the top part of Figure 7.4, MRI was more reliable than CT to describe the large volume and the diffuse spread of the lesions. Some cystic lesions are seen in contact with the mesentery and in contact with the bowel loops with a diffuse enhancement on the post-contrast images.

On CT, the nodular aspect is seen but it is not so easy to be sure that the lesions are not resectable. Because of extensive tumor deposits at the junction of small bowel with its mesentery (Figure 7.4 bottom), the surgeon only performed a large debulking but not a complete cytoreduction.

The radiologist also has to describe the number and the location of the stenosis of small bowel segments as well as colonic or gastric invasion. In the patient shown in Figure 7.5, only two stenoses were depicted on CT as well on PET-CT. In fact, at surgery there were five different bowel obstructions and the patient was not resectable because the sacrifice of the small bowel was too extensive.

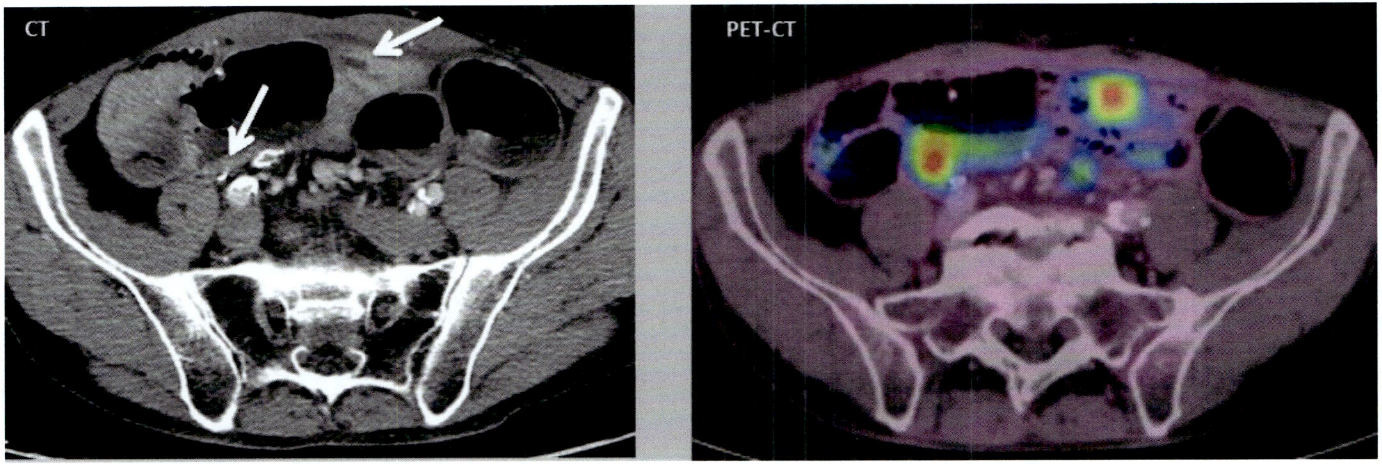

Figure 7.5. Peritoneal lesions secondary of a gastric cancer causing constriction of the small bowel (arrows).

Diffuse involvement of the root of the mesentery also has to be described, including the relationship of the lesions with the mesenteric vessels. In the patient of Figure 7.6, the diffuse nodular infiltration of the whole mesentery was obviously non-resectable with evident retraction of the mesenteric root.

Another site is the hepatoduodenal ligament involvement as shown in Figure 7.7. It is not so easy to describe an unresectable lesion in this anatomic location, unless there is obvious biliary or vascular stenosis. In Figure 7.7, all the radiologists who performed the three different exams failed to describe an unresectable lesion in the hepatoduodenal ligament. They saw that there was a lesion but they did not pay attention to its exact location. The patient had open and close surgery because of this infiltration. A radiologic concerning feature is the partial or complete disappearance of the fatty tissue within the hepatoduodenal ligament. This may be seen well in pseudomyxoma, but it also occurs in other primary tumors [6]. In colorectal cancer, changes in the liver hilum usually indicates an unresectable lesion (Figure 7.8). In fact, retrospectively one can see a partial disappearance of the fat as a consequence of infiltration within the tissue of the portal triad.

The third site is the pelvis with unresectable lesions that may correspond to diffuse or frozen pelvis, or bladder and trigone involvement. Regarding trigone involvement, MRI is the technique of choice because in the absence of bilateral hydroureter, it will be very difficult to see on CT or on PET-CT [7]. The ureters are not always involved (Figure 7.9). Involvement of the trigone usually precludes cytoreductive surgery, as the patient is unlikely to have a complete surgery unless extreme resections are performed (cystectomy).

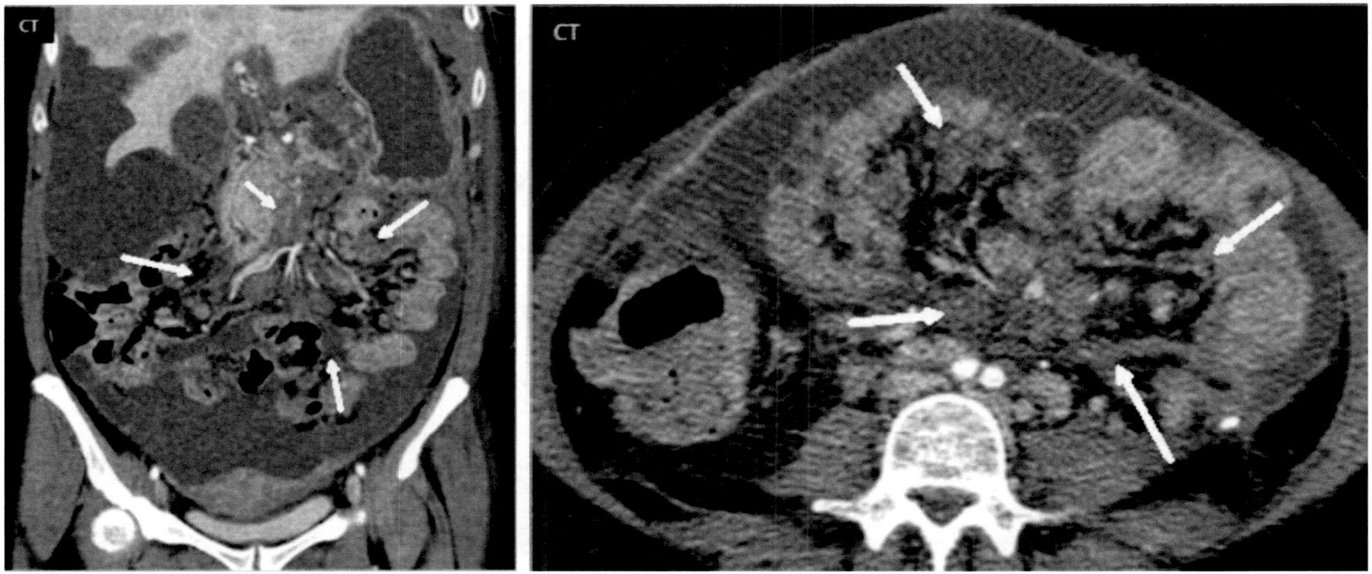

Figure 7.6. Diffuse involvement of the root of the mesentery (arrows) in a patient with colorectal cancer.

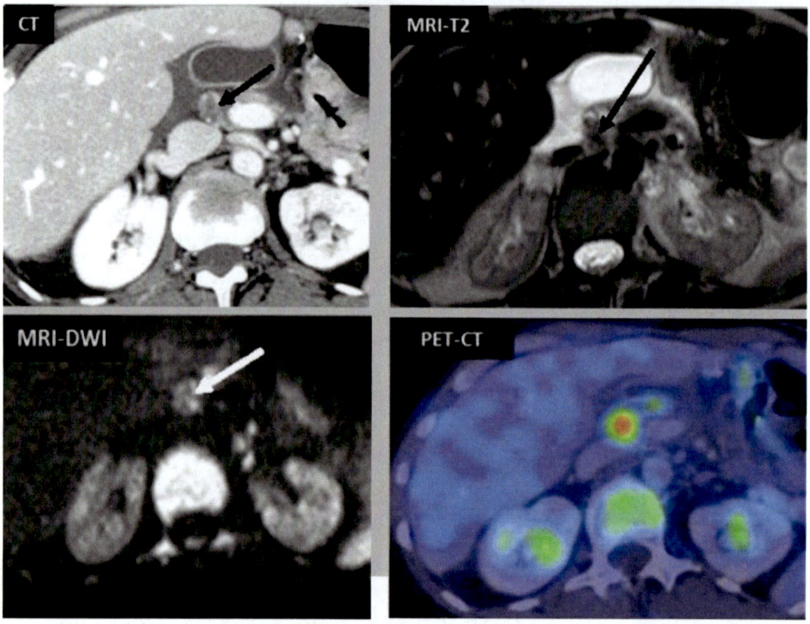

Figure 7.7. Lesions from a colorectal cancer in the hepatoduodenal ligament (arrows) may be unresectable. If a cytoreduction is attempted an open and close surgery may result.

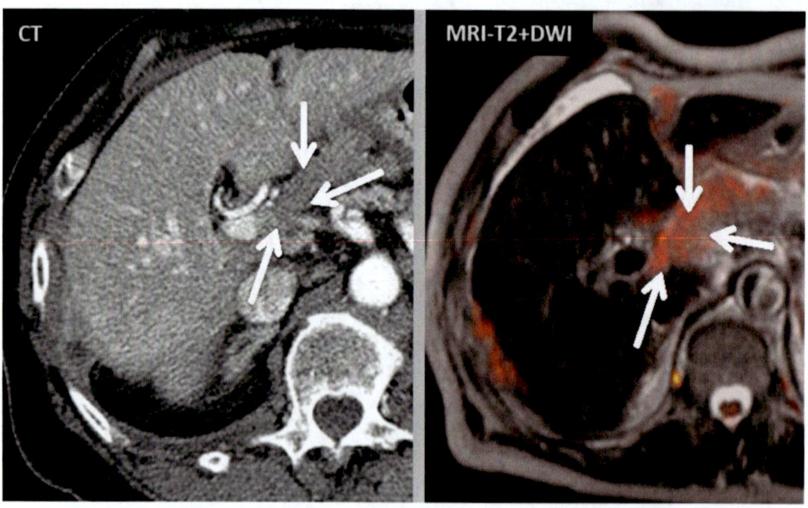

Figure 7.8. In this colorectal cancer patient, partial disappearance of the fat in the hepatoduodenal ligament (arrows) was a result of cancer infiltration. There was an open and close surgical procedure.

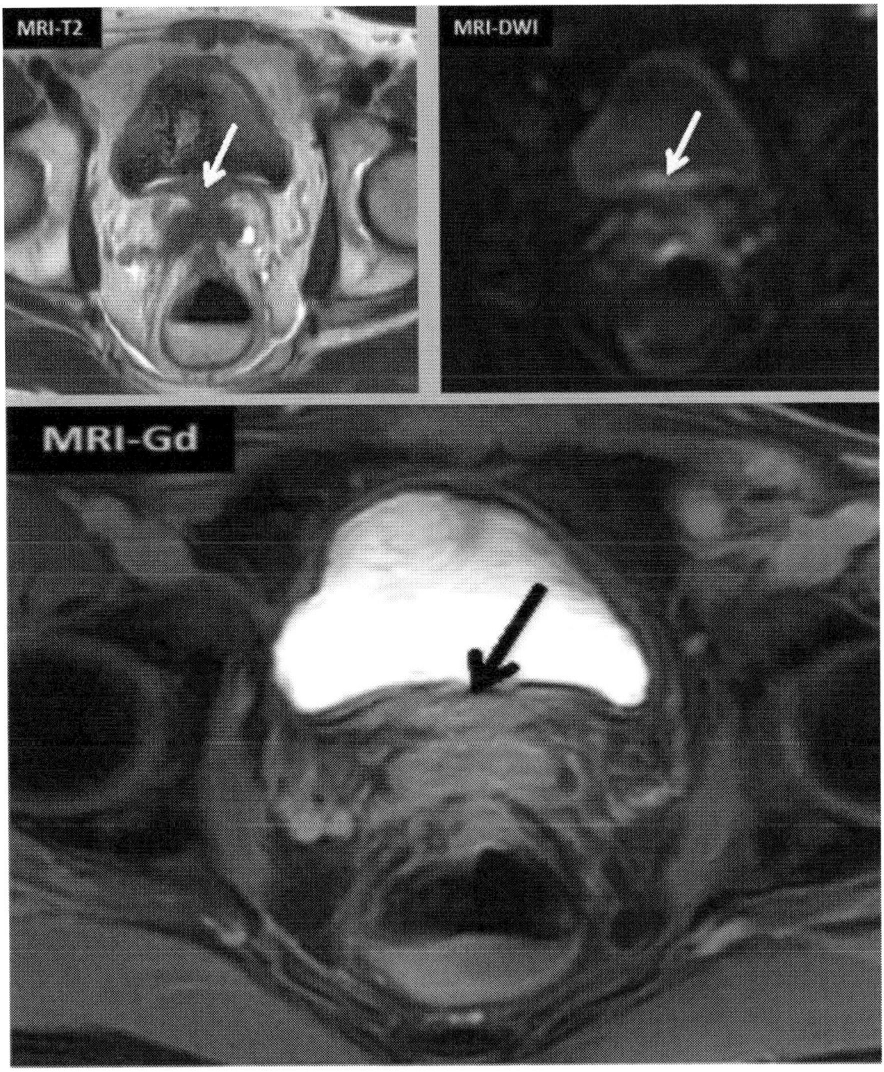

Figure 7.9. Trigone involvement (arrows) without bilateral ureteral obstruction in a patient with colorectal cancer.

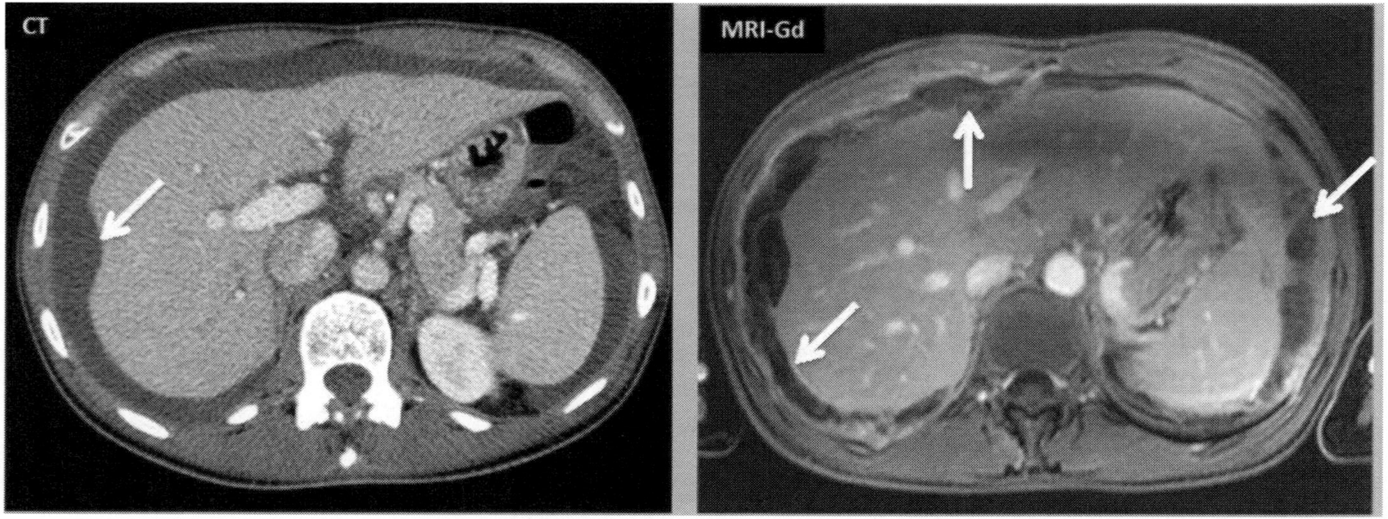

Figure 7.10. Subphrenic tumor deposits (arrows) that required extensive peritonectomy for their complete removal in a patient with pseudomyxoma. The extent of the lesion is better seen on MRI.

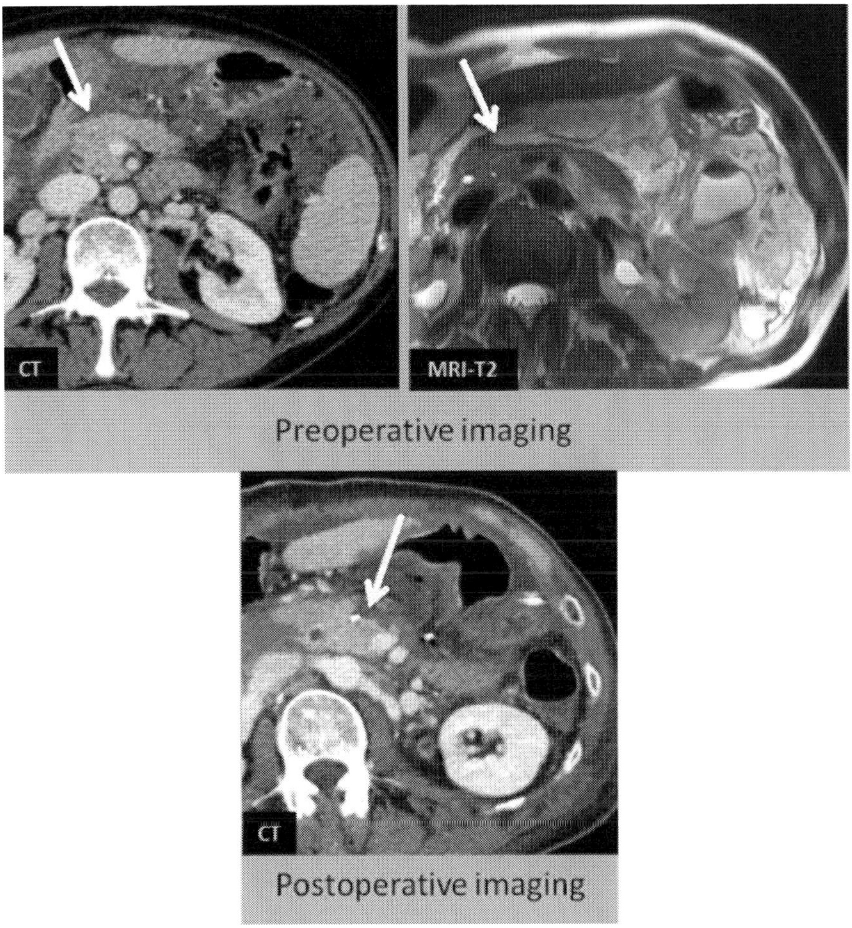

Figure 7.11. Preoperative imaging by CT and MRI-T2 of peritoneal metastases on the anterior peritoneal surface of the pancreas (arrows). Postoperative CT shows a metal clip (arrow) at the site from which the tumor deposit was removed.

Detection of Lesions of the Anatomic Site That Require Surgical Subspecialty Expertise

The second type of lesion the radiologist has to describe in the qualitative radiologic analysis are those that will require special surgical expertise for resection because they are at a difficult anatomic site [1]. Due to surgical progress, most of the parietal peritoneal lesions are technically resectable but some are associated with a higher morbidity and mortality. The radiology report must describe the type and the number of such lesions.

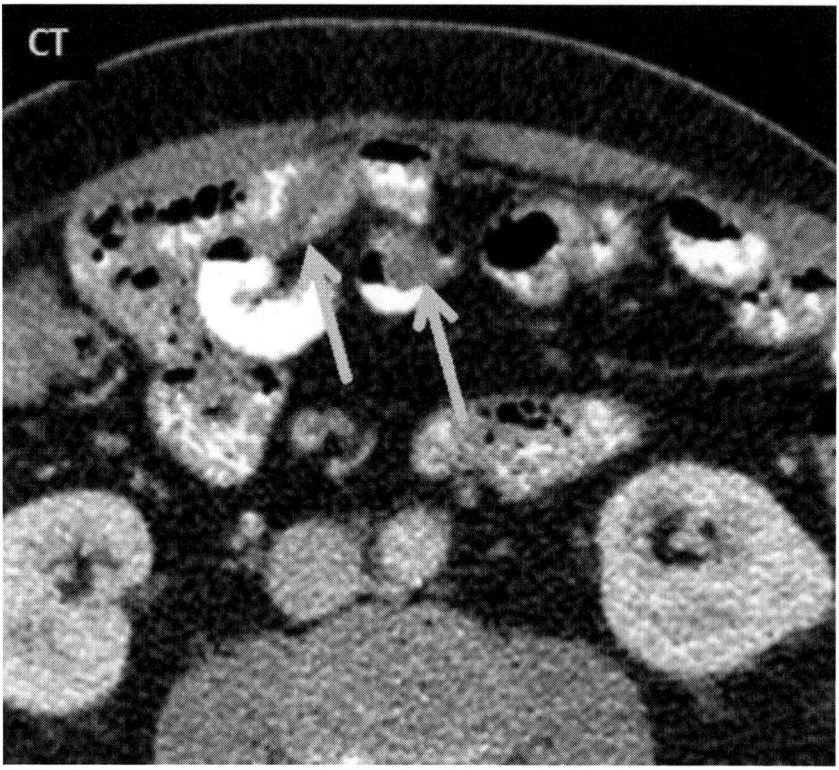

Figure 7.12. Peritoneal metastases from a colorectal cancer associated with the small bowel (arrows) and its mesentery. Bowel resection will be required.

All of these features have to be presented in the multidisciplinary consultation meeting. Indeed, as previously said, while a single concerning radiologic feature will often add complexity to the cytoreductive surgery, two or more concerning radiologic features usually indicates a suboptimal resection and/or add morbidity that has to be taken into account [3-5]. These lesions are:

1. Diffuse spread of liver capsule or of diaphragm. For example, report of extensive perihepatic involvement requires particular surgical skill for removal using extensive glissonectomy. The lesion depicted in Figure 7.10 would also require left and right subphrenic peritonectomy to achieve the optimal surgical outcome. The surgeon has to remove all the lesions by performing peritonectomy.
2. Peri-pancreatic lesions, pyloric or duodenal obstruction. The pancreas is an organ that carries high surgical morbidity because the capsule is friable. A higher risk of leakage of pancreatic enzymes occurs with any surgical trauma. Radiologists not only have to describe lesions in the lesser sac but also describe the relationships with the pancreas. In Figure 7.11, well displayed on the MRI on T2 image is a scalloping and even a notch on the pancreas surface, better seen than on CT. The surgeon performed a complete resection. On the postoperative CT the presence of a clip in the notch was present.
3. Multifocal lesions of mesentery, one or two small-bowel stenosis, diffuse involvement of colon. Bowel resection requires more extensive procedures and is problematic because of anastomotic leakage. The location as well as the number of the lesion on the mesentery, the small bowel, the large bowel, and also the stomach have to be described. In Figure 7.12, numerous nodules in the mesentery are depicted and at surgery the surgeon was required to perform extensive small bowel resection.
4. Encasement of one ureter and/or involvement of urinary bladder dome, or seminal vesicles,

5. Pelvic sidewall and vascular spaces (external iliac vessels).
6. Muscular involvement (psoas, abdominal wall).

Detection of Occult Peritoneal Metastases

The third type is the hidden lesion that the surgeon may fail to visualize on routine exploration. Some surgeons say, "what the surgeon doesn't see may kill the patient." Such a lesion can be in ligaments, as in Figure 7.13 top. This figure shows a lesion in the deep part of the falciform ligament. The lesion was reported by the radiologist but unfortunately the surgeon missed it. In follow-up, a clip around the lesion is seen on CT but the lesion was still there and has grown (Figure 7.13 bottom).

Hidden lesion can also be in the spleen and deeply imbedded (Figure 7.14). Sometimes the lesion develops more in the subperitoneal space than at the surface of the peritoneum. If associated adhesions cover the nodule, the surgeon may miss it. In this context, the functional imaging may be very useful to better display these nodules (Figure 7.15).

Sometimes there are very hidden lesions for surgeons because lesions are in the retroperitoneal space. There may be communication and opening into this space as a result of previous surgery, but there is also congenital communications between the peritoneal cavity and the retroperitoneal space. In Figure 7.16, a very small nodule is located in behind the hepatorenal recess or Morrison's pouch. If the surgeon is not alert to inspect this anatomic site, he won't see it.

In Figure 7.17, there is a lesion in the abdominal wall as a result of the extrinsic infiltration at a laparoscopy port site or biopsy site.

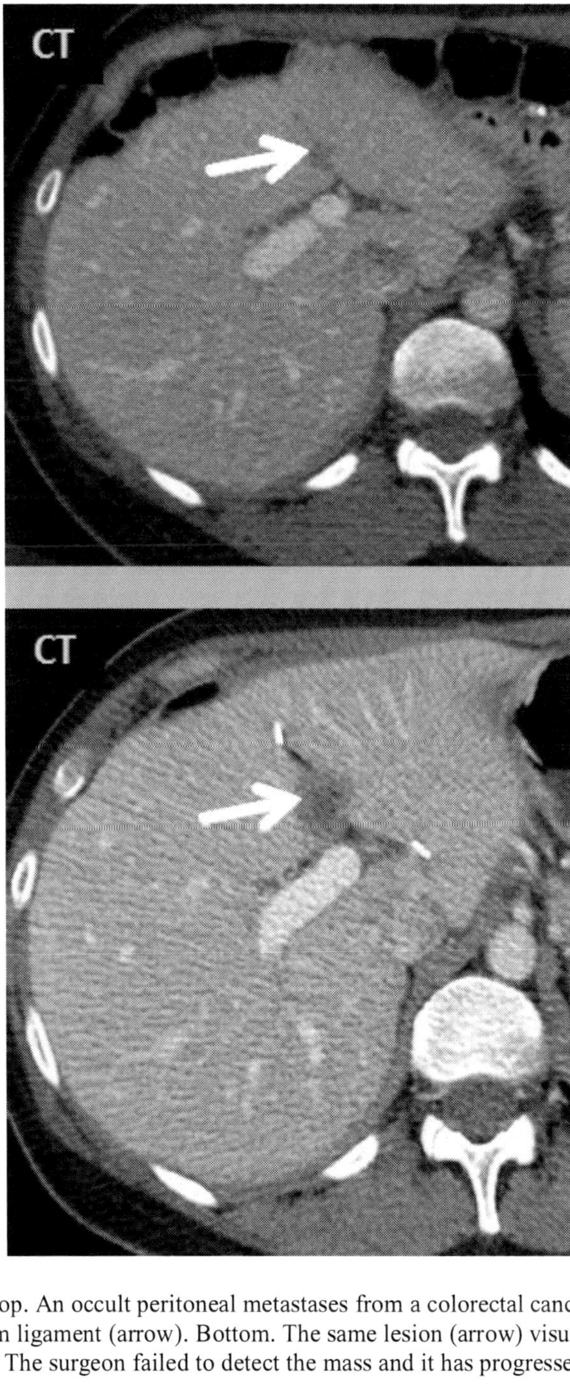

Figure 7.13. Top. An occult peritoneal metastases from a colorectal cancer hidden deep to the falciform ligament (arrow). Bottom. The same lesion (arrow) visualized on follow-up CT. The surgeon failed to detect the mass and it has progressed.

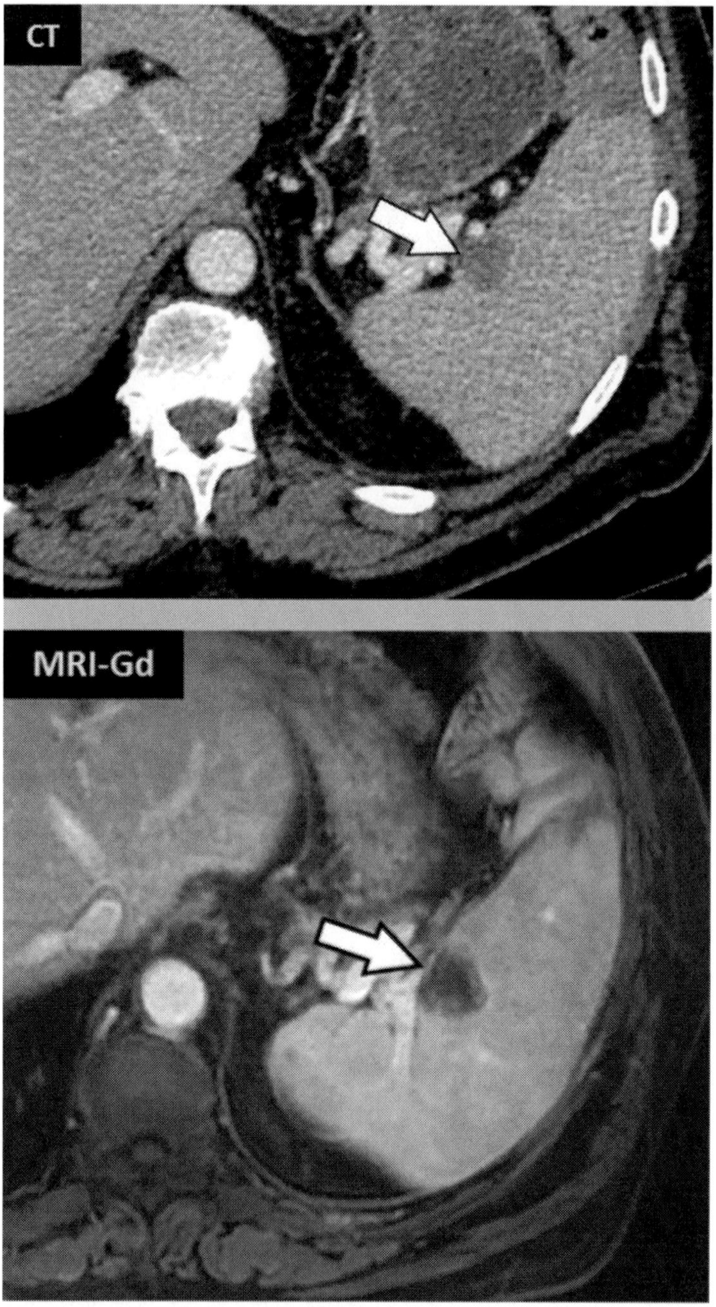

Figure 7.14. Top and bottom. CT and MRI-Gadolinium that shows a lesion deep within the hilum of the spleen (arrows) in a patient with colorectal cancer.

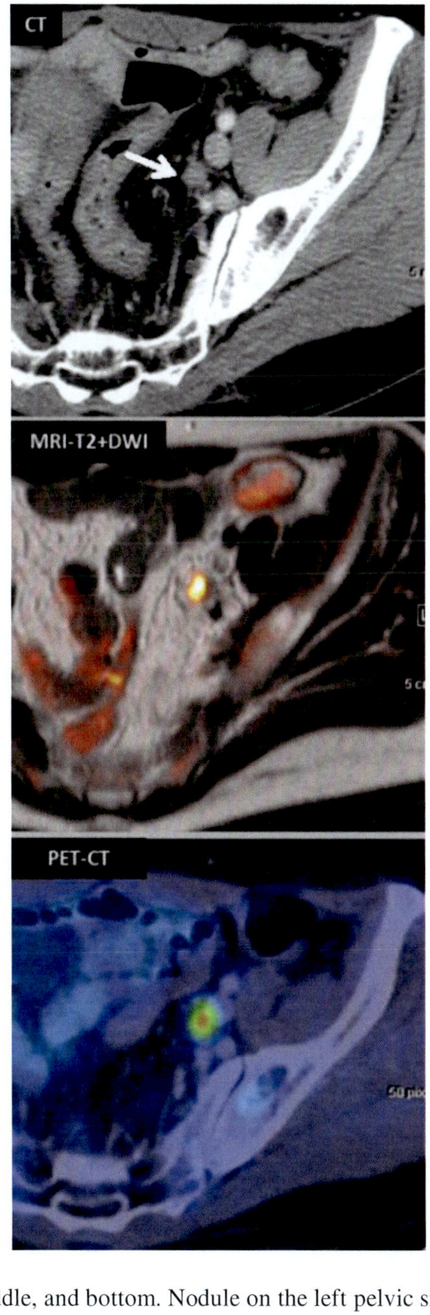

Figure 7.15. Top, middle, and bottom. Nodule on the left pelvic sidewall (arrow) covered by an adhesive process in a patient with ovarian cancer. Lesion was more subperitoneal than on the surface.

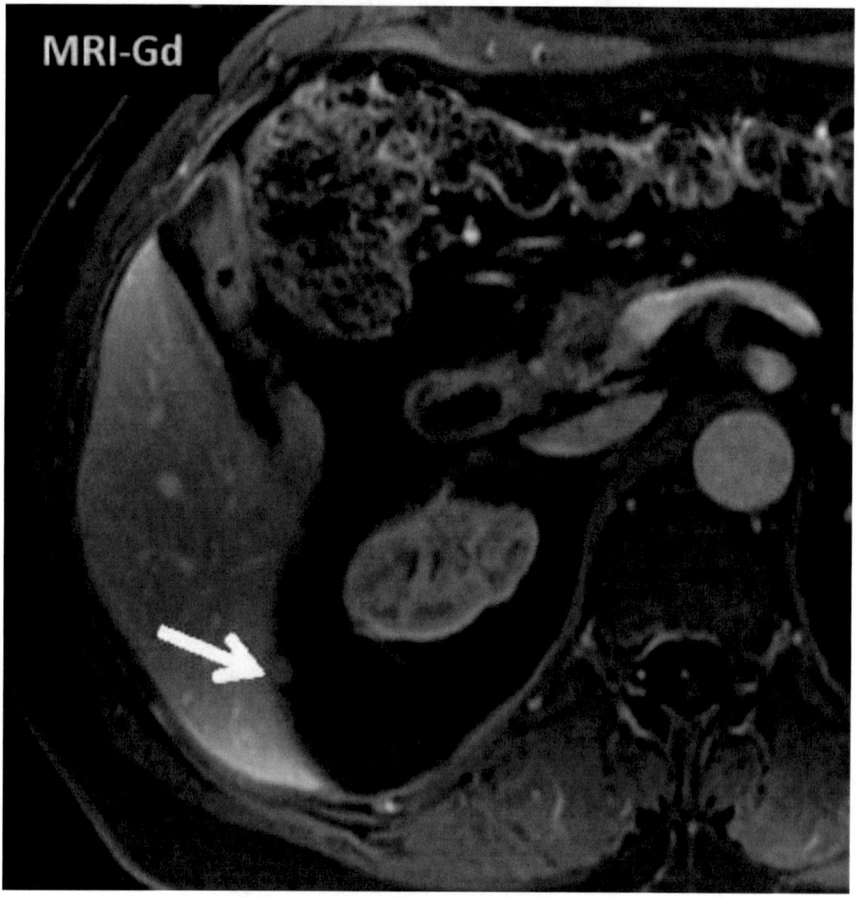

Figure 7.16. Peritoneal metastases deep within Morrison's pouch (arrow) in a patient with colorectal cancer.

Sometimes, the radiologist is called upon to describe the lesions not accessible at laparoscopy, for example, in the lesser sac, the Morisson pouch or the posterior aspect of the liver (Figure 7.18). This is all the more important when a laparoscopic approach is chosen to perform cytoreduction and HIPEC in benign cystic mesothelioma or low grade PMP with small tumor volume. If the radiologist identifies some lesions in blind spots at laparoscopy, the surgeon has to choose to do the laparotomy.

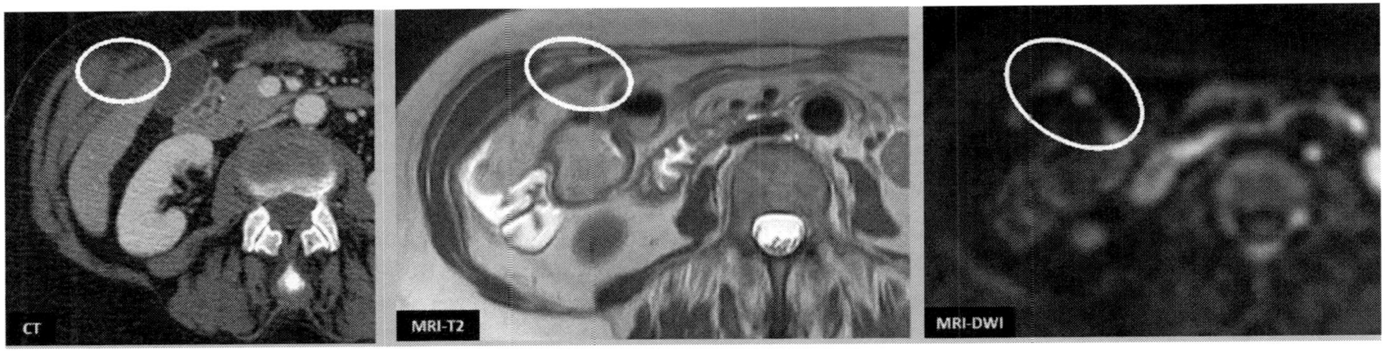

Figure 7.17. A lesion in the abdominal wall (circles) initially unseen by CT but well depicted by MRI-T2 and MRI-diffusion weighted image.

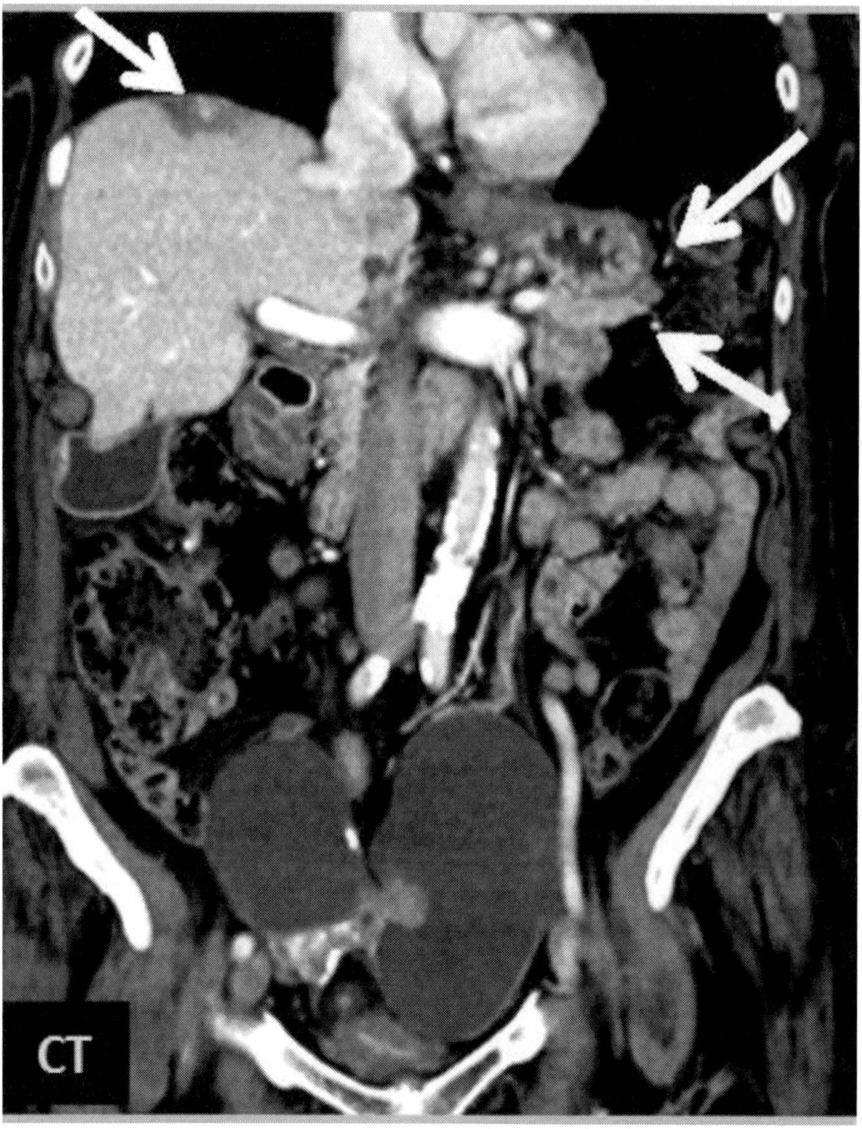

Figure 7.18. Lesions from ovarian cancer not visible by laparoscopy may be on the posterior aspect of the right lobe of the liver or within the lesser sac (arrows).

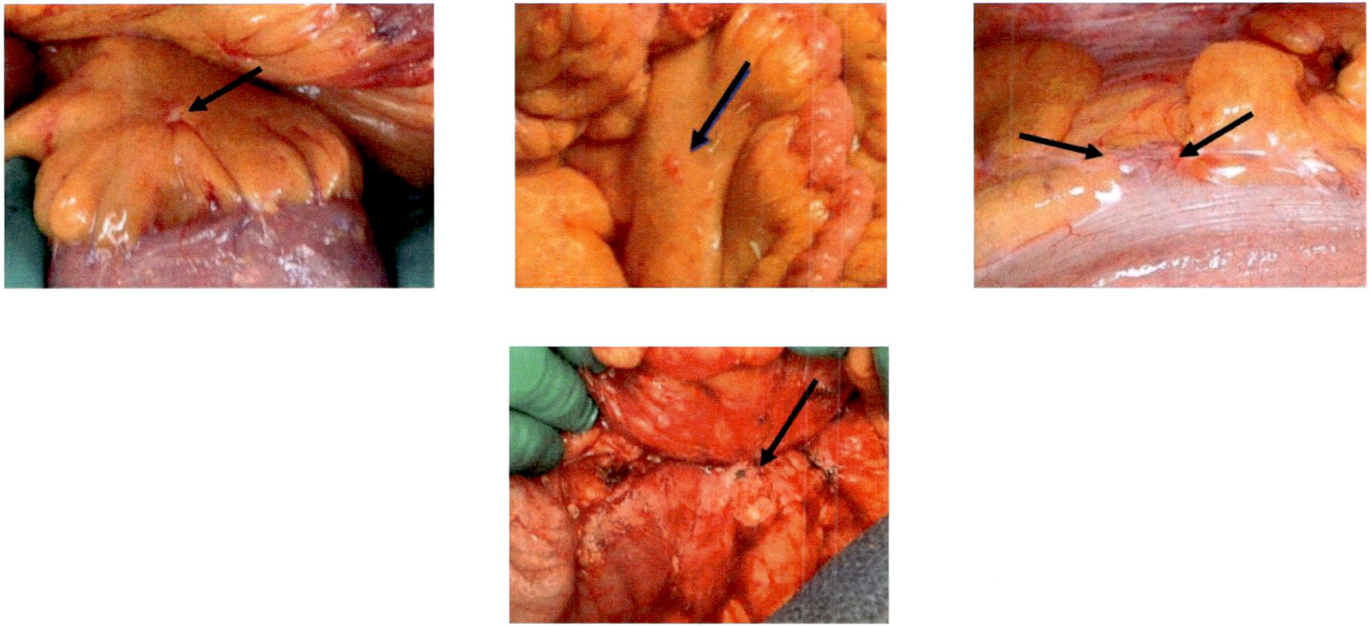

Figure 7.19. These very small peritoneal metastases (arrows) (left and middle), as well as plaque like lesion (arrows) (right) or tumor adhesion (arrow) (bottom) are readily visible by the surgeon but invisible by radiology.

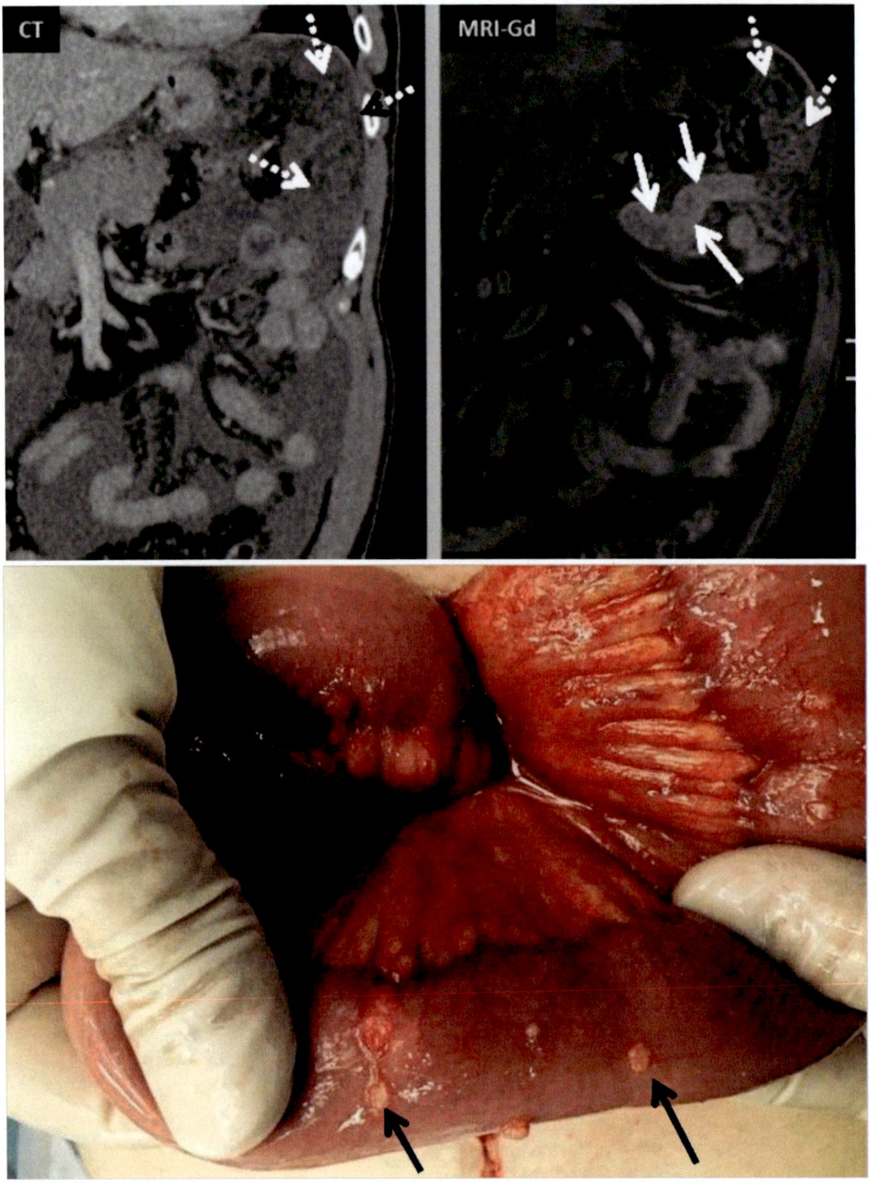

Figure 7.20. Top. The peritoneal lesions shown are overestimated as lesion size 3 (>5 cm) on radiologic peritoneal cancer index with an extensive peritoneal thickening and fat stranding of greater omentum (dashed arrows) by CT and MRI and consequent serosal enhancement of jejunal loops by MRI only (arrows). Bottom. The mesothelioma nodules of the bowel serosa (arrows) are visualized at surgery as peritoneal cancer index size 1 (0-2.5 mm).

THIRD STEP: QUANTITATION BY A RADIOLOGIC PERITONEAL CANCER INDEX (PCI)

The third step required in the written report for a peritoneal metastases patient is a quantitative analysis. This is the very challenging radiologic peritoneal cancer index (PCI) [8, 9]. All studies have the same conclusion – CT, and often MRI, completely underestimate the PCI [10-14]. Even when radiologists think they are correct and have the same PCI score of the surgeon, often one finds a region that is overestimated with false positive, or underestimated in some region. Although, it is thus very difficult, the radiological PCI can be made more accurate using MRI or even by combining CT and MRI compared with CT alone [15,16, 17].

The most common cause of underestimation is the small or thin lesion. The very small lesions shown in Figure 7.19 are readily visible by the surgeon but difficult for the radiologist and usually invisible at imaging.

In contrast, as a result of peritoneal thickening and fat stranding radiologists overestimate some lesions. In Figure 7.20 top, there is enhancement of the serosa of the jejunum. It's more than 5 cm so it should be scored as radiologic PCI lesion size of 3. But when surgeon looked at the bowel surface there were only very tiny lesions and the surgeon gave a lesion size score of 1. Probably there is some inflammation and the enhancement is due more to the inflammation than the nodule. Another difficulty is to know how to score fat stranding. It can have several different causes. Sometime the surgeon will palpate a huge infiltration of the fat tissue but, sometimes only small nodules at the surface are present and the fat stranding is due to lymphatic blockage. Sometimes he feels nothing and it is only ascites. Fat stranding is thus very difficult to score. To improve the radiological PCI, a comprehensive and accurate radiological lexicon is needed to provide a score that strongly correlates the radiological and surgical findings.

Although a radiologic PCI is difficult, radiologist should still make the effort to calculate the radiologic PCI for several reasons. First, it standardizes the radiological reading. Second, it forces the radiologist to screen every lesion and give an estimate regarding the extent and distribution of the peritoneal metastases. Third, it provides an idea of the tumor volume. The estimate of tumor distribution is perhaps more informative than the exact numerical value of the PCI. Finally, it may also help evaluate the response to neoadjuvant chemotherapy. The response criteria are not usually available in peritoneal metastases as they are often non-target lesions.

At a minimum, the radiologist should provide a semi-quantitative assessment, describing if the spread is diffuse, multifocal or localized, and to report the number of regions involved out of 13.

Fourth Step: Description of Extraperitoneal Metastases

The fourth step necessary to provide a written report for a peritoneal metastases patient is to describe extraperitoneal metastases. Depending on the site and the number, it can dramatically change the management of the patient. For liver, spleen, pleural or osseous metastases, CT, MRI, or PET-CT can be used depending on the primary tumor. In Figure 7.21, the osseous lesion in the rib precluded surgery.

Regarding lymph nodes, PET-CT is the technique of reference for detection and characterization whatever the location of the lymph nodes. In the retroperitoneum, above or under the renal pedicle, in the celiac region, in the mesentery, or even in the extra-abdominal region, PET-CT is indicated (Figure 7.22).

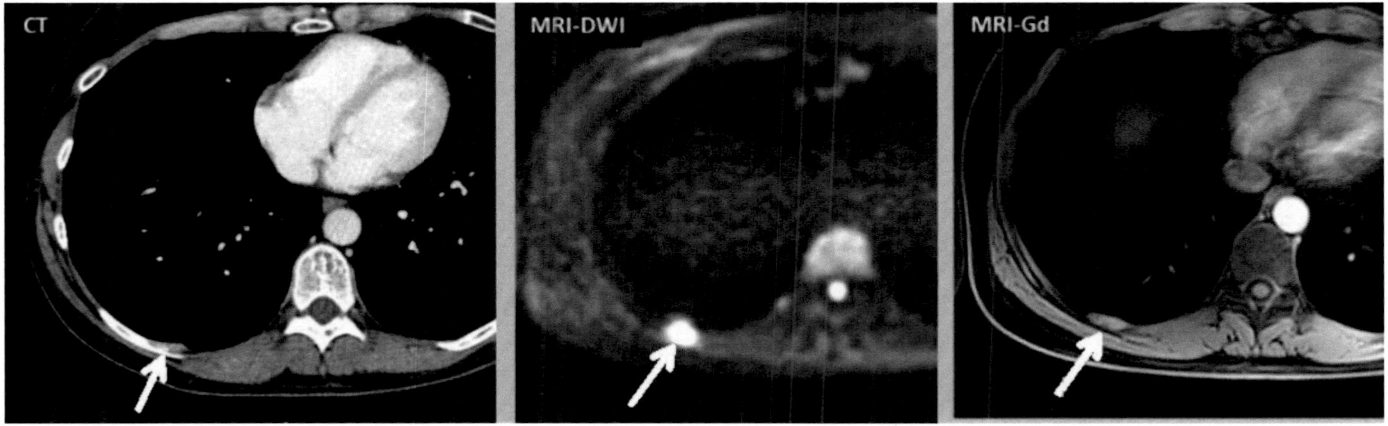

Figure 7.21. Osseous metastases (arrows) of a colorectal cancer that profoundly affected patient management decisions.

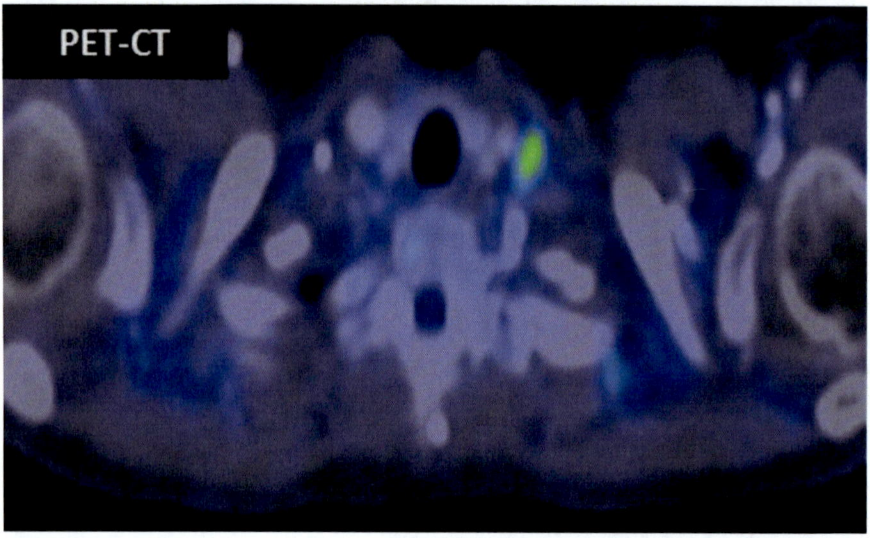

Figure 7.22. Identification of extraperitoneal metastases. A left supraclavicular lymph node by PET-CT that was suspect and biopsy positive in a patient with ovarian cancer.

Fifth Step: Search for the Primary Cancer

As a final step in construction of a written report for patients with peritoneal metastases, the radiologist must search for a primary cancer. Particularly when unknown, the radiologist has to perform an extraperitoneal analysis with dedicated reading to find the primary cancer or guide the clinician for management in tertiary referral center if needed (Figure 7.23). A clue for rare primary peritoneal disease, peritoneal mesothelioma for example, is the absence of a primary gastrointestinal or gynecologic malignancy.

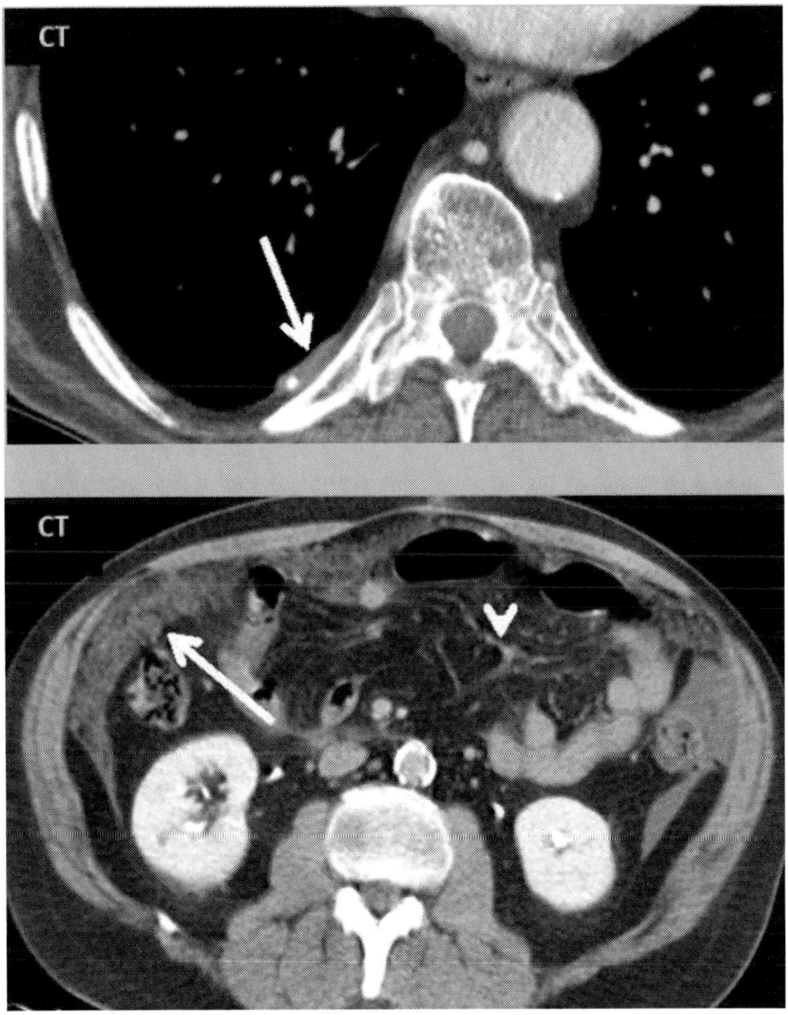

Figure 7.23. Top. Presence of a pleural plaque partially calcified (arrow) suggestive of asbestos exposure. Bottom. Presence of unspecific peritoneal metastases with greater omentum infiltration (arrow) and mesenteric thickenings (arrowhead) with no predominant primary site suggests malignant peritoneal mesothelioma as a primary malignancy.

Use of Peritoneal Malignancy Stage Evaluation – PROMISE

Because this radiologic evaluation of peritoneal metastases is not simple, an internet free application called PROMISE as been created by the expert center of Lyon Sud University Hospital (France). PROMISE for PeRitOneal MalIgnancy Stage Evaluation is available at the internet address, www.e-promise.org [18]. The software facilitates tabulation and automatically calculates PCI and other surgically validated scores. It offers computer-assistance to produce a quick, very precise and standardized pre-, intra-, or post-operative reports of the extent of the peritoneal metastases. It also may help to specialize non-specialized institutions in their current practice and facilitate research in multicenter studies on peritoneal surface malignancy. Data can also be exported in an Excel database that can be then loaded on a radiologist's computer for research or translational research.

Table 7.1. A minimal and standardized radiology report for peritoneal metastases

- Presence or absence of peritoneal metastases
- Qualitative analysis
    - Concerning radiologic features indicate potential unresectable lesions
    - Lesions that require surgical subspecialty expertise
    - Hidden lesions for the surgeon
- Quantitative analysis using PCI
- Presence of extraperitoneal metastases
- Search for the primary cancer (initial staging)

In conclusion, a minimal and standardized report has to be provided by the radiologist to optimize the multidisciplinary management of patients with peritoneal metastases. The 5 steps in constructing an optimized report of peritoneal metastases are 1) determine presence or absence of peritoneal metastases, 2) construct a qualitative analysis describing three types of lesions: potential unresectable lesions, lesions that require surgical subspecialty expertise for resection, and hidden lesions that the surgeon may miss, 3) quantitative analysis using PCI, 4) establish the presence versus absence of extraperitoneal metastases, 5) finally, there should always be a search for a primary cancer site, particularly in initial staging (Table 7.1).

REFERENCES

[1] Sugarbaker PH, van der Speeten K. An overview of peritonectomy, visceral resection, and therapeutic laparoscopy for peritoneal surface malignancy. (In) Sugarbaker PH (Ed). Cytoreductive Surgery & Perioperative Chemotherapy for Peritoneal Surface Malignancy. Textbook and Video Atlas. 2nd Edition. *Cine-Med Publishing*: Woodbury, CT, 2017, pp. 17-46.

[2] Rivard JD, Temple WJ, McConnell YJ, Sultan H, Mack LA. Preoperative computed tomography does not predict respectability in peritoneal carcinomatosis. *Am J Surg* 2014;207:760-765.

[3] Sugarbaker PH, Sardi A, Brown G, Dromain C, Rousset P, Jelinek JS. Concerning CT features used to select patients for treatment of peritoneal metastases, a pictoral essay. *Int J Hyperthermia* 2017;33(5):497-504.

[4] Jacquet P, Jelinek JS, Chang D, Koslowe P, Sugarbaker PH. Abdominal computed tomographic scan in the selection of patients with mucinous peritoneal carcinomatosis for cytoreductive surgery. *J Am Coll Surg* 1995;181:530-538.

[5] Yan TD, Haveric N, Carmignani P, Chang D, Sugarbaker PH. Abdominal computed tomography scans in the selection of patients with malignant peritoneal mesothelioma for comprehensive treatment with cytoreductive surgery and perioperative intraperitoneal chemotherapy. *Cancer* 2005;15:839-849.

[6] Menassel B, Duclos A, Passot G, et al. Preoperative CT and MRI prediction of non-resectability in patients treated for pseudomyxoma

peritonei from mucinous appendiceal neoplasms. *Eur J Surg Oncol.* Apr 2016;42(4):558-566.

[7] Cotton F, Pellet O, Gilly FN, Granier A, Sournac L, Glehen O. MRI evaluation of bulky tumor masses in the mesentery and bladder involvement in peritoneal carcinomatosis. *Eur J Surg Oncol* 2006;32(10):1212-1216.

[8] Jacquet P, Sugarbaker PH. Current methodologies for clinical assessment of patients with peritoneal carcinomatosis. *J Exp Clin Cancer Res* 1996;15(1):49-58.

[9] Harmon RL, Sugarbaker PH. Prognostic indicators in peritoneal carcinomatosis from gastrointestinal cancer. *Int Semin Surg Oncol* 2005;2(1):3.

[10] Jacquet P, Jelinek JS, Steves MA, Sugarbaker PH. Evaluation of computer tomography in patients with peritoneal carcinomatosis. *Cancer* 1993;72(5):1631-1636.

[11] de Bree E, Koops W, Kroger R, et al. Peritoneal carcinomatosis from colorectal or appendiceal origin: correlation of preoperative CT with intraoperative findings and evaluation of interobserver agreement. *J Surg Oncol* 2004;86:64-73.

[12] Koh JL, Yan TD, Glenn D, Morris DL. Evaluation of preoperative computed tomography in estimating peritoneal cancer index in colorectal peritoneal carcinomatosis. *Ann Surg Oncol* 2009;16:327-333.

[13] Esquivel J, Chua TC, Stojadinovich A, et al. Accuracy and clinical relevance of computed tomography scan interpretation of peritoneal cancer index in colorectal cancer peritoneal carcinomatosis: A multi-institutional study. *J Surg Oncol* 2010;102:565-570.

[14] Sala E, Kataoka M, Pandit-Taskar N, et al. Recurrent ovarian cancer: use of contrast-enhanced CT and PET/CT to accurately localize tumor recurrence and to predict patients' survival. *Radiology* 2010;257(1):125-134.

[15] Low RN, Barone RM, Lucero J. Comparison of MRI and CT for predicting the Peritoneal Cancer Index (PCI) preoperatively in

patients being considered for cytoreductive surgical procedures. *Ann Surg Oncol.* 2015 May;22(5):1708-1715.

[16] Dohan A, Hoeffel C, Soyer P, et al. Evaluation of the peritoneal carcinomatosis index with CT and MRI. *Br J Surg. Aug* 2017;104(9):1244-1249.

[17] van 't Sant I, van Eden WJ, Engbersen MP, Kok NFM, Woensdregt K, Lambregts DMJ, Shanmuganathan S, Beets-Tan RGH, Aalbers AGJ, Lahaye MJ. Diffusion-weighted MRI assessment of the peritoneal cancer index before cytoreductive surgery. *Br J Surg*. 2018 Oct 24. doi: 10.1002/bjs.10989.

[18] Villeneuve L, Thivolet A, Bakrin N, Mohamed F, Isaac S, Valette PJ, Glehen O, Rousset P; A new internet tool to report peritoneal malignancy extent. PeRitOneal MalIgnancy Stage Evaluation (PROMISE) application. BIG-RENAPE and RENAPE Working Groups. *Eur J Surg Oncol.* 2016 Jun;42(6):877-882.

In: Pictorial Essays … ISBN: 978-1-53618-014-5
Editors: PH Sugarbaker and RN Low ©2020 Nova Science Publishers, Inc.

Chapter 8

In 100 Patients with Malignant Peritoneal Mesothelioma, Concerning CT Features Predicted Outcome of Treatment

James S. Jelinek, MD
Department of Radiology, MedStar Washington Hospital Center,
Washington, DC, US

Introduction

At a consensus conference of the Peritoneal Surface Oncology Group International (PSOGI) in Milan in December 2006 the CT of abdomen and pelvis was determined to be the standard radiologic test to which all others should be compared [1]. Recent studies have shown that multiparametric MRI, using gadolinium and diffusion-weighted imaging, is more accurate than CT in determining a preoperative PCI in patients being considered for HIPEC [2, 3]. At most institutions, CT remains the first radiologic test for these patients [4]. As early as 1995, Jacquet and coworkers showed that CT was valuable in the selection of patients with mucinous peritoneal metastases for cytoreductive surgery. Sixteen parameters were analyzed and six were determined to be useful for predicting the outcome of surgery [5]. Yan and coworkers performed a similar study in 30 patients who had cytoreductive surgery for malignant peritoneal mesothelioma. Thirty-nine CT parameters were described and statistically analyzed to determine their association with adequate versus suboptimal cancer resection. They reported that the combination of a tumor mass greater than 5 cm in the epigastric region and loss of architecture of the small bowel regions had a 100% likelihood of suboptimal cytoreduction [6]. Rivard et al. studied seven concerning CT features in 15 patients with peritoneal metastases who had cytoreductive surgery. One concerning CT feature did not predict suboptimal cytoreduction but two correlated significantly with a poor surgical outcome [7]. Recently, Sugarbaker and coworkers published a pictoral essay that evaluated the utility of preoperative CT to assess prognosis in patients with a variety of diseases causing peritoneal metastases. They described 15 concerning CT features and the anatomic pathology with which these images were associated [8]. These concerning features were presented as a consensus regarding CT evaluation of peritoneal metastases patients with several gastrointestinal or gynecologic malignancies.

The data in our current manuscript takes these concerning CT features beyond the prior studies. Prior reports correlated CT features with the outcome of surgery, usually complete versus incomplete cytoreduction. Now the concerning CT features in patients being evaluated for initial treatment of malignant peritoneal mesothelioma are correlated with the survival of these patients treated uniformly with cytoreductive surgery plus intraoperative hyperthermic intraperitoneal chemotherapy (HIPEC). To our knowledge this is the first attempt to quantitatively evaluate the pretreatment CT findings and correlate them with overall survival.

PATIENTS AND METHODS

All peritoneal mesothelioma patients who had surgical treatment at this institution were entered into a prospective database. From the current study patients with sarcomatoid, biphasic, cystic, and papillary histologies were excluded. All of the epithelial malignant peritoneal mesothelioma patients who had a preoperative CT available for review were entered into this study. The initial intervention at this institution was cytoreductive surgery as described elsewhere [9]. In all patients the surgical intervention was accompanied by HIPEC [10]. All patients received 6 cycles of neoadjuvant or adjuvant chemotherapy with pemetrexed and cisplatin. Patient follow-up was a 6 monthly visit to a surgeon or medical oncologist for symptom review and physical examination for 3 years and then yearly for another 7 years. A CT scan with oral and intravenous contrast was performed at the same intervals. Follow-up was often performed by the referral institution.

Survival was prospectively obtained from the patient or referring physician. Permission from the institutional review board to collect and analyze data on these malignant peritoneal mesothelioma patients was obtained.

COMPUTED TOMOGRAPHY SCANS

Because the current study was performed over a 22-year time period, a variety of CT scanners and protocols were utilized. Also, some CTs were obtained from a referral institution. For all patients, there was a minimum 1-cm continuous slice thickness through the entire chest, abdomen and pelvis. The radiologic studies were performed after the administration of oral and intravenous contrast media. All of the CT scans were read by a staff radiologist and these findings included in the data in this manuscript. For the current clinical research study, all CT scans were reread by a single radiologist and single surgeon to determine concerning CT features. The initial group of concerning CT features were those described by

Sugarbaker et al. [8]. As the review of these preoperative CTs were studied other images that would qualify as a concerning CT feature for malignant peritoneal mesothelioma were added and evaluated. The physicians were aware that all patients in the study had clinical evidence of malignant peritoneal mesothelioma and were to be treated at this institution.

In order to be included in this study, a malignant peritoneal mesothelioma patient had a CT performed within two weeks prior to the surgical intervention available for critical evaluation regarding concerning CT features. In three patients who had neoadjuvant chemotherapy, the CT prior to the initiation of systemic treatments was used.

As a comparison for the utility of this radiologic assessment to predict outcome, objective assessment of the prognostic value of extent of disease came from the peritoneal cancer index (PCI) [11]. This assessment determines the size of peritoneal nodules in 13 abdominal-pelvic regions with the abdomen open at the time of cytoreductive surgery. The score ranges from 0 (no visible disease) to 39 (tumor nodules greater than 5 cm in all 13 abdominal-pelvic regions). To assess the prognostic value of the extent of cancer resection by cytoreductive surgery, the completeness of cytoreduction (CC) score was used. This assessment measures the largest nodule or layer of cancer in 13 abdominal-pelvic regions that remains after the best efforts at cytoreductive surgery. No visible disease was scored as CC-0. CC-1 indicated all nodules or layers are less than 0.25 cm, CC-2 nodules from 0.25 to 2.5 cm and CC-3 greater than 2.5 cm [11].

STATISTICAL ANALYSIS

To evaluate the radiologic findings, the official radiologic interpretations were reviewed. Then a surgeon and radiologist again studied the CT with special concern to identify additional concerning radiologic features present preoperatively and relevant to malignant peritoneal mesothelioma.

Initially all concerning CT features were evaluated and scored as present versus absent. The percentage of patients with a particular concerning CT feature was determined. Then the survival was determined for a particular group with a concerning CT feature present as compared to the concerning CT feature absent. These data were statistically analyzed with univariate survival analysis to compare the survival time between groups of each CT feature. As a secondary analysis, the impact of none, one, or two or more concerning CT features on survival was determined using a Kaplan-Meier survival analysis. Multivariate Cox proportional hazard regression was modeled to assess simultaneously the effect of all concerning CT features on survival time. The model pooled all CT features that were found significant in univariate survival analysis plus the number of CT features and determined a set of factors that remain a significant contribution after adjusting each other. The impact of PCI and CC score on these patients were presented as a comparison for the concerning CT features survival analysis.

RESULTS

Patient Characteristics

From the database of 165 peritoneal mesothelioma patients, 100 were identified as eligible for this study. All patients had biopsy confirmed malignant epithelial peritoneal mesothelioma, a preoperative CT available for review, treatment with an initial cytoreductive surgery plus HIPEC and follow-up until date of death or until October 1, 2019. The PCI and CC score were available for all 100 patients. There were 57 males. Ages ranged from 21 to 74 with a median of 51. The patient data and CT scans were accumulated since 1998.

Formulating a List of Concerning CT Features for Malignant Peritoneal Mesothelioma

Our first effort was to determine the presence versus absence of the concerning CT features described in our previous manuscript [8]. In the current study our initial assessment established that some of the concerning CT features identified in peritoneal metastases patients from multiple primary sites were not present in peritoneal metastases patients undergoing their initial treatment. Also, an accurate CT-PCI, as previously described, was not possible because of the CT technology available over the 22 years these CT scans were accumulated. None of our malignant peritoneal mesothelioma patients showed retroperitoneal or mesenteric lymphadenopathy, hydroureter, psoas muscle invasion, pelvic sidewall invasion, or gastric outlet obstruction. The two separate features, infiltration of the porta hepatis and mass greater than 5 cm in the greater omentum, were not clearly distinguishable in these malignant peritoneal mesothelioma patients and so were combined as a single concerning CT feature [8].

Six Concerning CT Features Previously Described

Six concerning CT features retained from the original list were assessed on all 100 patients. Obstructed portions of the small bowel were present in 7% of patients. An example of obstructed small bowel is shown in Figure 8.1. In this 36-year-old women, the bowel is markedly dilated with air. No transition site from dilated to normal caliber of bowel was present.

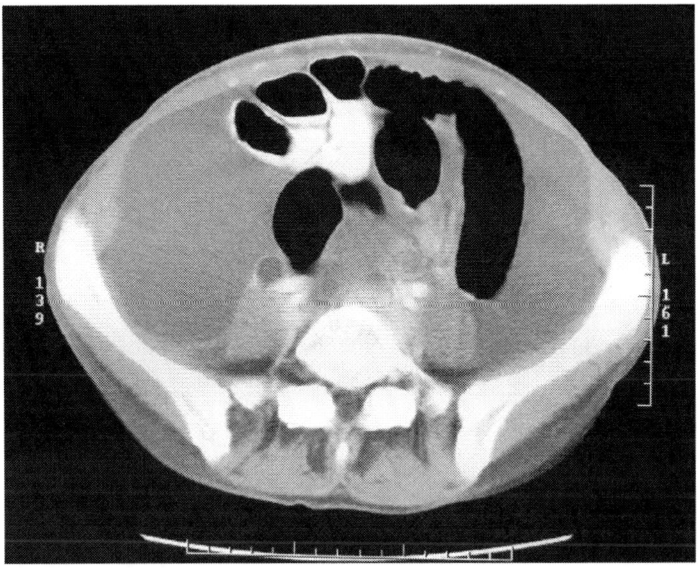

Figure 8.1. Obstructed bowel. The small bowel is dilated with increased quantities of air. Air fluid levels are infrequent and the obstruction was not complete in any patient.

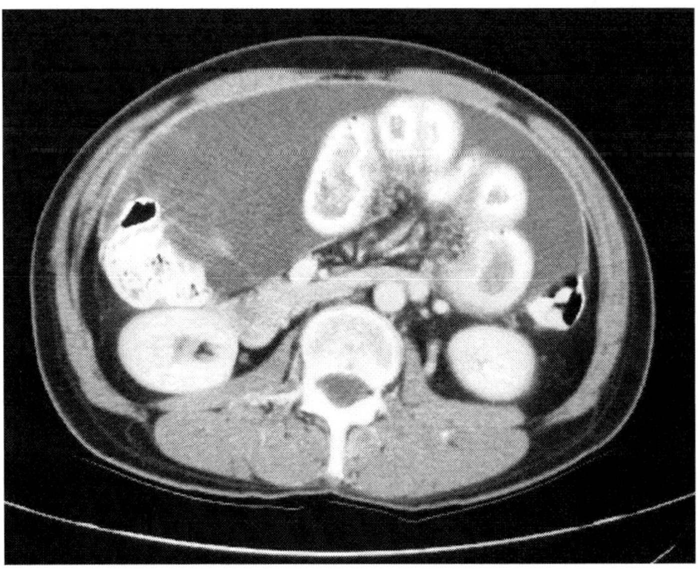

Figure 8.2. Clumped bowel. The mesentery of the small bowel is fixed and foreshortened by mesothelioma.

In 16% of patients, portions of the small bowel mesentery were retracted, referred to as clumped bowel. An example is illustrated in Figure 8.2. In this 52-year-old woman, the small bowel mesentery appeared foreshortened and fixed.

In Figure 8.3, the small bowel mesentery is infiltrated by tumor. In this 51-year-old man, the mesentery for the most part remains in its anatomic position but the space between the leaves of the mesentery are infiltrated by tumor. Tumor masses located between the leaves of small bowel mesentery were distinguished from ascites by differences in density. This difference was upon occasion subtle. The small bowel mesentery infiltrated by tumor was present in 41% of patients.

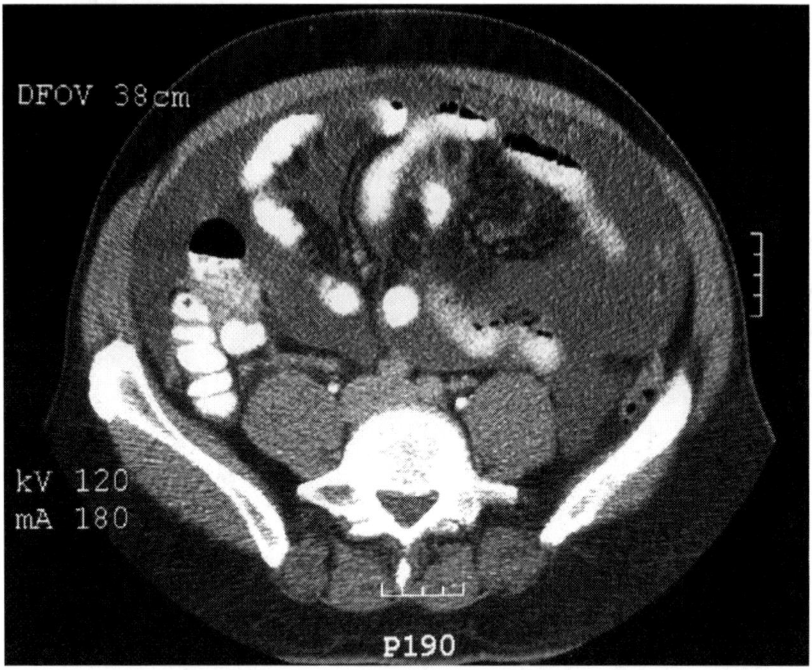

Figure 8.3. Small bowel mesentery infiltrated by tumor. The small bowel and its mesentery remain in their anatomic position. However, the space between the folds of the mesentery are infiltrated by mesothelioma.

If Figure 8.4, the deep pelvis is invaded by tumor. In this 28-year-old male, the seminal vesicles are not distinguishable from the mass of mesothelioma present within the pelvis. In a woman with prior hysterectomy, deep pelvic invasion by mesothelioma is indicated by tumor infiltrating the apex of the vagina. If the uterus is present, a tumor mass and not ascites fills the pelvis. The deep pelvis infiltrated by tumor was reported in 21% of patients.

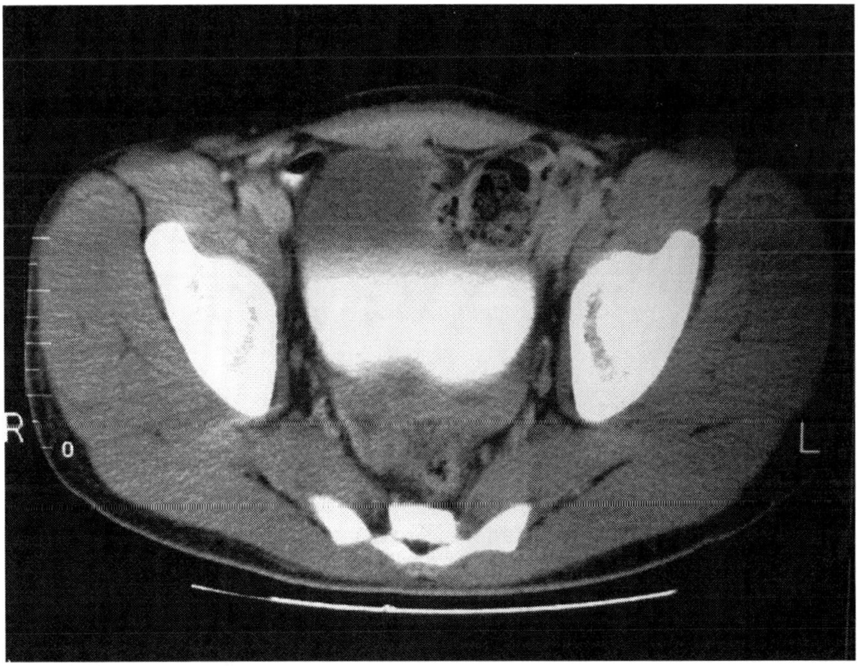

Figure 8.4. Deep pelvis invaded by tumor. The seminal vesicle in this male patient (or apex of vagina in a female) were not distinguishable from the mass of pelvic mesothelioma.

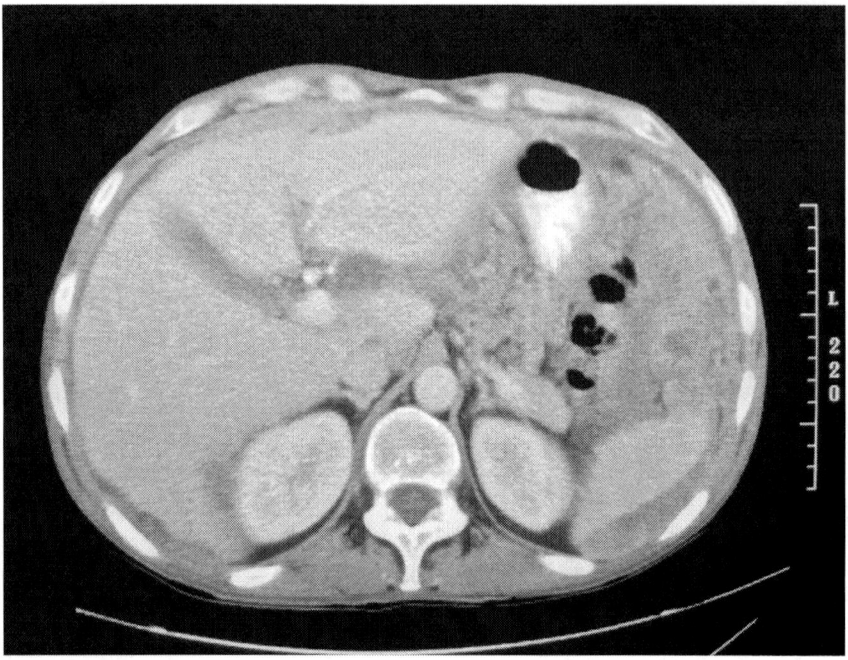

Figure 8.5. Infiltration of the porta hepatis and/or lesser omental mass greater than 5 cm. Mesothelioma infiltrates and surrounds the structures of the porta hepatis and is contiguous with tumor external to the liver.

For this study of the CT in malignant peritoneal mesothelioma, infiltration of the porta hepatis and a lesser omental mass greater than 5 cm were coexistent features. They were present in 15% of patients. In Figure 8.5, this 23-year-old woman had mesothelioma infiltration into porta hepatis contiguous with a tumor mass within the lesser omentum.

In 15% of patients, a tumor mass greater than 5 cm was immediately adjacent to the proximal jejunum. No bowel obstruction was seen but the mass effect was obvious in this 52-year-old man. A mass greater than 5 cm contiguous with the proximal jejunum was seen in 16% of these patients (Figure 8.6).

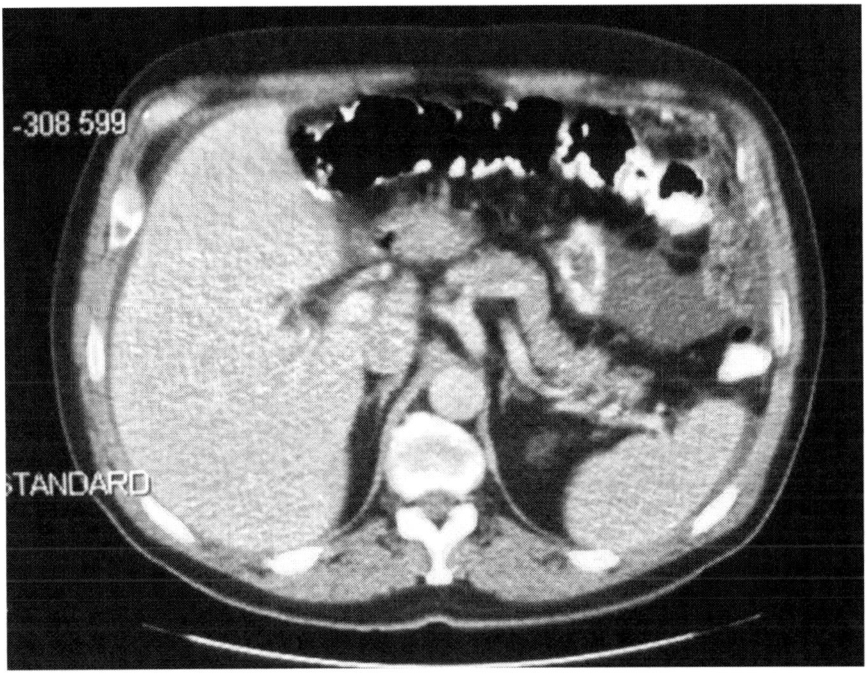

Figure 8.6. Mass greater than 5 cm adjacent to the jejunum.

Five Concerning CT Features Specific for Malignant Peritoneal Mesothelioma

As a result of the preliminary study of CT scans from these 100 patients, five new concerning CT features not listed in our prior publication were added to the preoperative evaluation of malignant peritoneal mesothelioma [8]. Pleural effusion was seen in 16% of patients. Pleural effusion was recorded as a concerning CT feature even if the amount of fluid was minimal. In Figure 8.7, the pleural fluid in this 37-year-old woman was minimal.

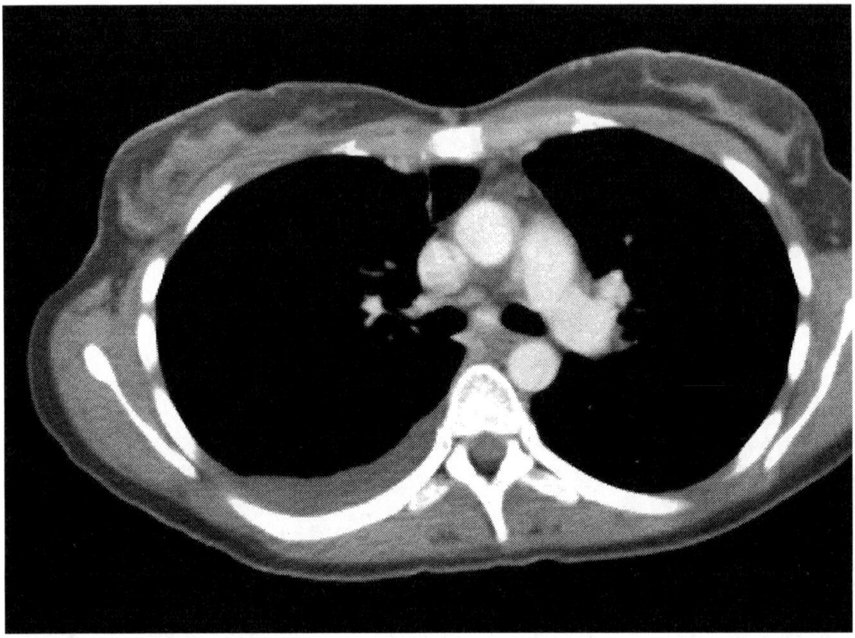

Figure 8.7. Pleural effusion was recorded as positive even with minimal fluid.

Figure 8.8 shows an enlarged (greater than 1.0 cm) right cardiophrenic angle lymph node in a 70-year-old male. The lymph node was not resected at the time of cytoreductive surgery [12]. Cardiophrenic angle lymph nodes were seen in 24% of patients. They were recorded as present if unilateral or bilateral.

Omental infiltration by tumor was quantitated as 0 (absent), 1+ minimal infiltration, 2+ moderate infiltration of the entire omentum or 3+ causing expansion of the abdominal wall by the greater omentum as an "omental cake." The incidence of all omental infiltrations was 49%; patients who showed 2+ or 3+, omental infiltration was 29%. In Figure 8.9, this 23-year-old female patient was scored as having a 3+ (marked) omental infiltration.

Ascites was assessed as present versus absent and was also quantitated. Zero indicated ascites was absent; 1+ indicated a small volume of fluid isolated at one or several sites within the abdomen or pelvis. A score of 2+ indicated the ascites was present in all quadrants of the abdomen and 3+

indicated abdominal distention by ascites. Some ascites was present in 69% of patients and 2+ or 3+ ascites present in 43%. In Figure 8.10, this 62-year-old woman was scored as having 3+ (marked) ascites.

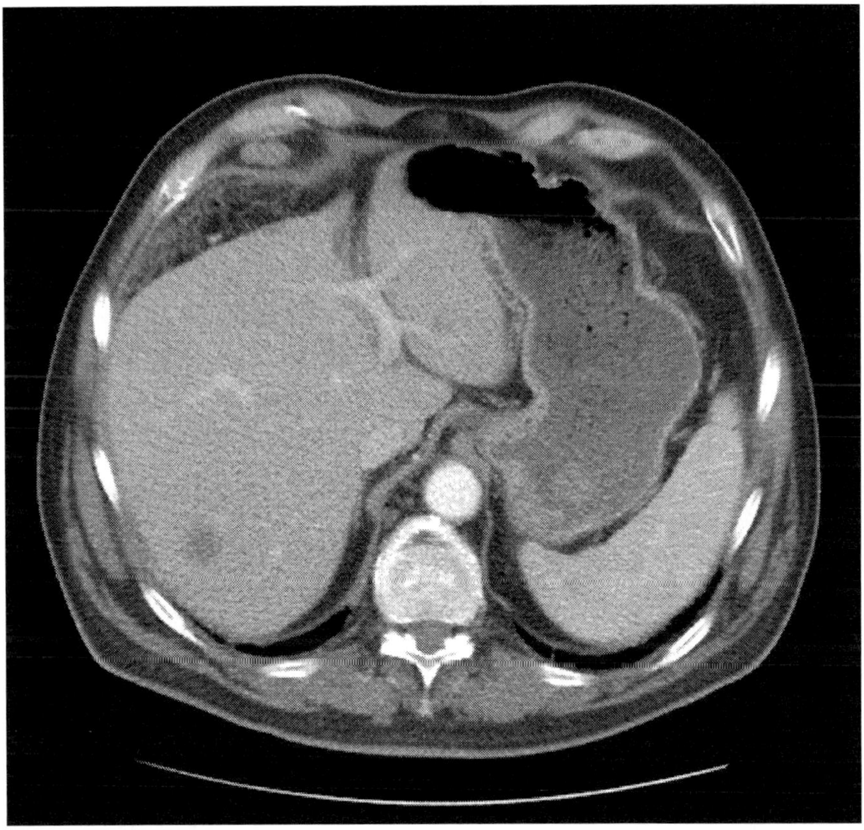

Figure 8.8. Enlarged cardiophrenic lymph nodes greater than 0.6 cm.

A final new concerning CT feature was a tumor mass greater than 5 cm within the peritoneal space but not adjacent to the jejunum. An isolated peritoneal mesothelioma mass was present in 5% of patients. The mass shown in Figure 8.11 was present in a 28-year-old man.

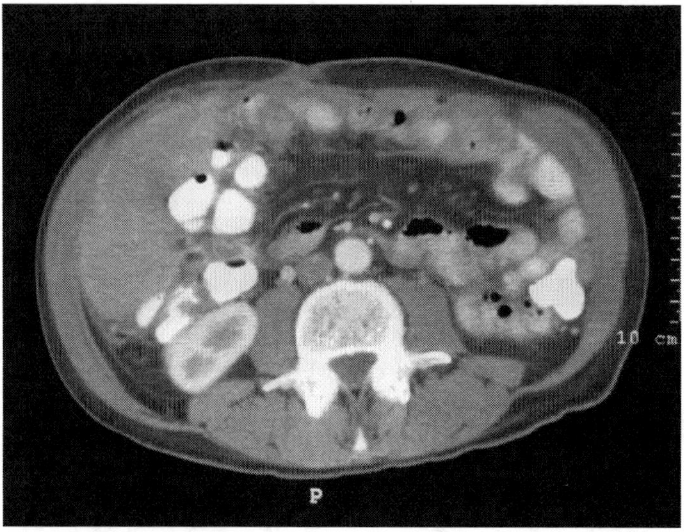

Figure 8.9. Omental infiltration was quantitated as 0, 1+, 2+ or 3+. A 3+ or marked infiltration is shown.

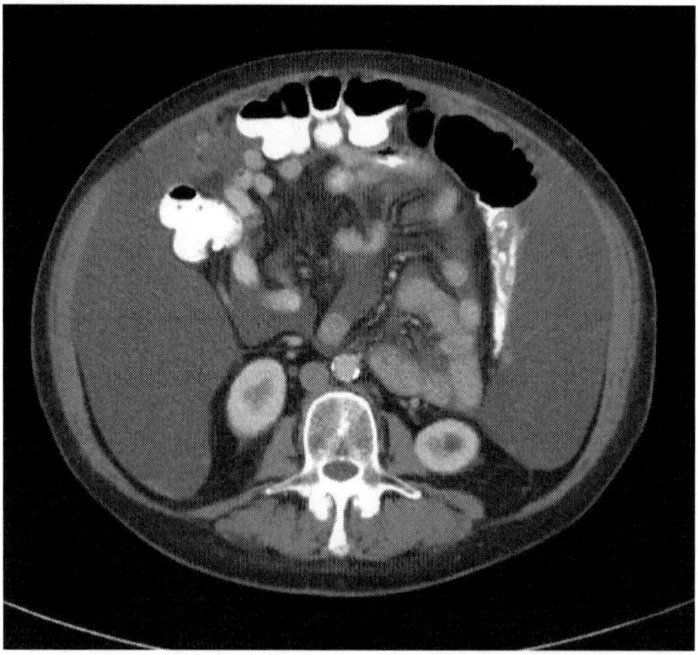

Figure 8.10. Ascites was quantitated as 0, 1+, 2+ or 3+. A 3+ ascites is shown.

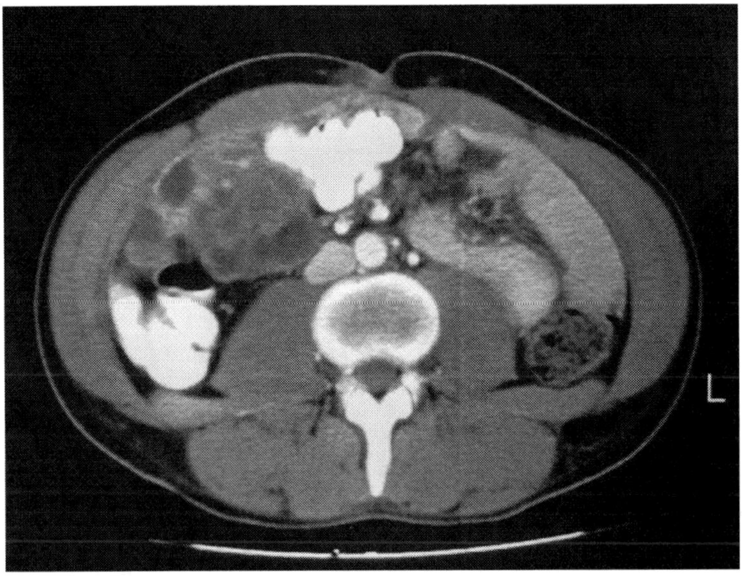

Figure 8.11. Tumor mass greater than 5 cm within the peritoneal space but not adjacent jejunum.

Table 8.1. Eleven concerning CT features and their preoperative evaluation in 100 patients with malignant peritoneal mesothelioma

Concerning CT feature	Incidence (%)	Median Survival (months) present/not present	Hazard Ratio (95% CI)	P-value
Obstructed small bowel	7	20/74	3.93 (1.73, 8.95)	0.0011
Clumped small bowel mesentery	16	17/82	3.13 (1.69, 5.80)	0.0003
Mesentery infiltrated	41	25/101	2.74 (1.65, 4.55)	0.0001
Deep pelvis invaded	21	17/74	2.04 (1.14, 3.68)	0.0173
Infiltrated porta hepatis and/or >5 cm mass in lesser omentum	15	25/74	2.04 (1.10, 3.79)	0.0230
Mass >5 cm adjacent jejunum	15	38/82	2.88 (1.58, 5.25)	0.0006
Pleural effusion	16	18/82	3.32 (1.86, 5.92)	<0.0001
Enlarged cardiophrenic angle lymph nodes	23	44/72	1.28 (0.71, 2.29)	0.4066
Omental infiltration 2+ and 3+	29	24/85	2.35 (1.40, 3.93)	0.0012
Ascites 2+ or 3+	43	25/101	2.66 (1.60, 4.42)	0.0002
Abdominal mass	5	39/72	1.64 (0.59, 4.53)	0.3391

In summary for each CT on these 100 patients there were 11 concerning CT features determined. Two of these CT features were quantitated (Table 8.1).

Analysis of Survival by Concerning CT Feature

For these 100 patients the survival estimate with number of patients at risk is shown in Figure 8.12. Median survival was 60 months. In Table 8.1, in addition to the percent of patients determined to show a particular radiologic feature, the median survival and hazard ratio of the group with the concerning CT feature present versus absent is indicated. Also, the statistical significance of the concerning CT feature on survival by univariate analysis is provided.

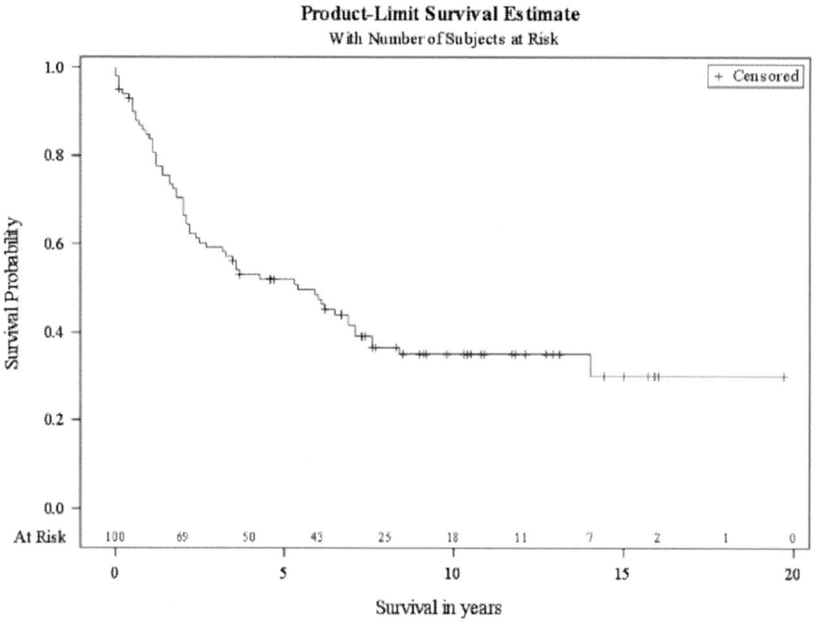

Figure 8.12. Survival estimate of 100 patients with malignant peritoneal mesothelioma with number of patients at risk.

Prognostic Impact of the Concerning CT Features

It is apparent from Table 8.1 that some concerning CT features had a more profound impact on prognosis than others. Seven of seven patients with obstructed small bowel failed the treatment. Fifteen of 16 patients in whom clumped small bowel mesentery was depicted died of this disease despite our aggressive treatments. Surprisingly pleural effusion, even if it was minimal, was associated with a poor outcome. In 16 patients with pleural effusion, 5 had a minimal amount of right pleural fluid. Fifteen of these 16 patients died of malignant peritoneal mesothelioma.

As a result of this analysis the presence of an enlarged cardiophrenic angle lymph node was not shown to have an impact on survival. Data regarding this CT feature was no longer considered a concerning CT feature and was not used in further survival analysis.

Comparison of Survival Estimates by Concerning CT Features, Peritoneal Cancer Index and Completeness of Cytoreduction Score

The three prognostic indicators available for malignant peritoneal mesothelioma patients are the concerning CT features, PCI and CC score. It is important to establish that the utility of those three parameters varies greatly in that the timing of the available information is very different. Concerning CT features provided statistically significant prognostic information preoperatively during the evaluation for cytoreductive surgery and HIPEC. In these 100 patients, 32 (32%) had no concerning CT features recorded. Fourteen (14%) had a single concerning CT features present and 54 (54%) had two or more concerning CT features ($p \leq 0.0001$). The Kaplan-Meier survival curve of these three groups of patients is shown in Figure 8.13. A peritoneal cancer index of 0-15 was compared to 16-30 versus greater than 30 ($p=0.0001$).

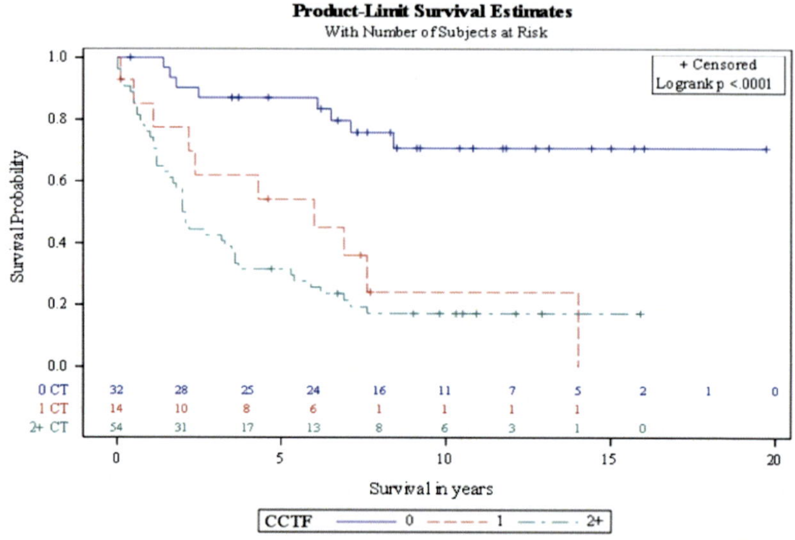

Figure 8.13. Survival by none versus a single versus two or more concerning CT features (CCTF) (p=<0.0001). Median survival of patients with no concerning features has not been reached. Median survival of patients with one CCTF was 82.4 months. For patients with 2 or more CCTF it was 24.3 months.

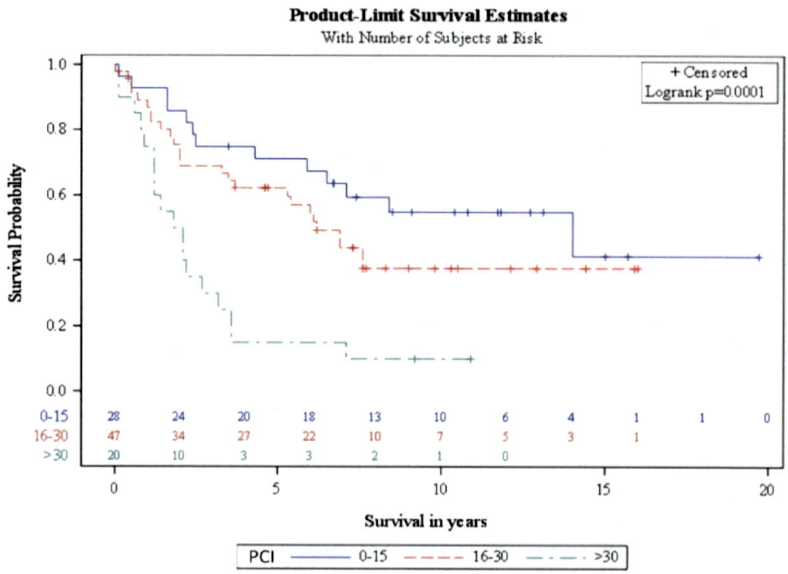

Figure 8.14. Survival by peritoneal cancer index (PCI) 0-15 versus 16-30 versus greater than 30 (p=0.0001).

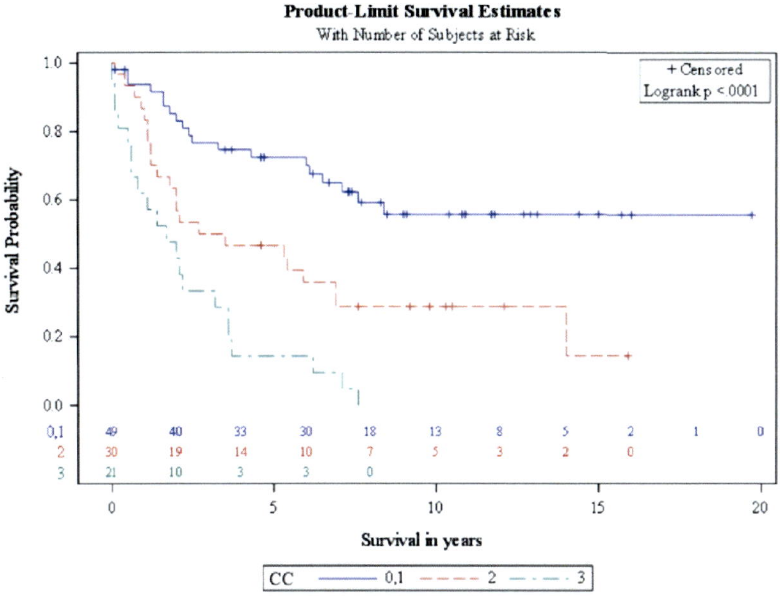

Figure 8.15. Survival by completeness of cytoreduction (CC) score 0 and 1 versus 2 versus 3 (p<0.0001).

This information was available for prognosis assessment at the time of surgical exploration for cytoreductive surgery. It is shown in Figure 8.14. Also, for comparison, the survival by completeness of cytoreduction score is shown in Figure 8.15. The graph shows survival in the completeness of cytoreduction 0 and 1 versus 2 versus 3 ($p \leq 0.0001$). This information was available for prognosis assessment only after the time the cytoreductive surgery was finished.

DISCUSSION

Concerning CT Features Provide an Assessment of Extent of Disease and an Estimate of Survival

Cytoreductive surgery plus HIPEC is currently the standard of care for patients with epithelioid malignant peritoneal mesothelioma [13]. This group of patients was treated by a standardized cytoreductive surgery and a standardized HIPEC treatment plan. With uniform treatment parameters it is a principle of cancer management that a smaller extent of disease is more successfully treated than advanced disease. Since malignant peritoneal mesothelioma is confined to the peritoneal space throughout its natural history, it is possible that CT can accurately determine the extent of disease and predict prognosis with treatment [14, 15]. This was the hypothesis with which this study was conducted. Our data shows that a greater extent of disease by CT as determined by the concerning CT features has a profound impact on survival. In the absence of concerning CT features, median survival was not available because more than 50% of patients with 0 concerning CT patients were still alive. With one concerning feature it was 82.4 months, and for 2 or more concerning features it was 24.3 months. These data had a p-value of <0.0001.

Although these CT concerning features are estimates of disease extent, it is possible that they also estimate the biology of the disease process. The radiologic characteristics that indicate tumor biology as more or less aggressive have not yet been described but may be important in an assessment of prognosis. The oncologist needs to be aware that some concerning CT features are associated with 100% likelihood of death from malignant peritoneal mesothelioma.

Additional Concerning CT Features

The concerning CT features that were tested for their impact on survival were not completely the same in this present study of malignant peritoneal mesothelioma patients as those listed in our initial publication [8]. In our initial survey of these 100 CTs, it became clear that additional specific CT features were important to assess in malignant peritoneal mesothelioma patients. Ascites was an obvious CT finding that may have prognostic implications in peritoneal mesothelioma patients but not in appendiceal mucinous neoplasm patients. Pleural effusion was a second added concerning CT feature. Omental infiltration was not thought to be prognostically important in appendiceal mucinous neoplasm patients but possibly had prognostic implications with peritoneal mesothelioma patients because of difficult dissection between transverse colon and greater omentum in this disease. We included omental infiltration as a concerning CT feature.

A fourth new concerning CT feature added was the presence of one or more enlarged cardiophrenic angle lymph nodes. The publications of Jeune et al. and Elias et al. suggested possible prognostic importance for this CT feature [12, 16]. Our data showed that enlarged cardiophrenic angle lymph nodes had no effect on outcome. This feature was eliminated from further analysis. A final new concerning CT feature was a mass greater than 5 cm in the peritoneal space. This new concerning CT feature was not shown to have negative prognostic implications (p=0.339). However, in our manuscript studying outcome with recurrence of peritoneal mesothelioma diagnosed in follow-up after cytoreduction and HIPEC treatment, a mesothelioma mass also had severe negative impact on prognosis [17]. The separate concerning CT feature of a mass greater than 5 cm adjacent to the jejunum was used as described in the prior manuscript [8].

The Current Assessment of Concerning CT Features Lacks More Sophisticated Radiologic Display

A deficiency of these data regarding perioperative CT is a lack of coronal and sagittal planes for imaging. The explanation comes from the radiologic technique available over the 22-year time period over which the study was conducted. Eighty of the 100 CT scans on individual patients were reconstructed on celluloid and only 20 originally printed digitally. In a majority of our clinical material only cross-sectional imaging was available. In order to maintain uniformity within our study, only cross-section images were used to generate these data. More sophisticated CT technique can be used for future studies that correlate CT images with prognosis in malignant peritoneal mesothelioma patients.

Incidence and Survival of Quantitated Concerning CT Features

It would be possible to quantitate many of the concerning CT features with modern CT technology now available. In this study the extent of ascites was quantitated as was the extent of omental infiltration. However, other concerning CT features such as mesenteric infiltration can be interpreted quantitatively [5]. The extent of pleural effusion could be quantitated although even a minimal effusion was associated with a poor outcome. The number of sites of bowel obstruction and the extent of foreshortening (clumping) of the small bowel mesentery could be quantitatively determined with sagittal and coronal images. In a preoperative radiologic evaluation, this quantitation might better assist in the selection of patients for an aggressive management plan rather than an assessment of present versus absent as in our present study. Also, other concerning CT features other than the 10 studied in this manuscript may be identified. In some patients, especially those with mucinous peritoneal metastases, MRI should be added to the preoperative radiologic evaluation [18].

Extent of Disease Predicts Prognosis Even though the Malignancy Is Resected

In studying colon cancer with peritoneal metastases, Gomez da Silva et al. showed that the extent of disease as measured by the peritoneal cancer index (PCI) is a robust indicator of prognosis even though all cancer is resected by a complete cytoreduction [19]. By the same principle the extent of disease as measured by CT may predict the outcome despite a complete removal by cytoreductive surgery plus HIPEC of malignant peritoneal mesothelioma. In peritoneal surface disease of minimal biologic aggressiveness such as the diffuse adenomucinosis (DPAM) of an appendiceal mucinous neoplasm, resection of an extremely large volume of tumor remains associated with a good prognosis [20]. However, with epithelioid type of malignant peritoneal mesothelioma, the outcome of treatment of the disease is less well correlated with complete resection. The biology of the disease process may be a major determinant of prognosis.

Comparison of the Utility of Concerning CT Features with the Other Established Assessments of Prognosis

It is not surprising that a greater extent of disease as determined by an increase in the peritoneal cancer index was correlated with a reduced prognosis. This has been demonstrated in the past by our own studies in malignant peritoneal mesothelioma and in the manuscripts from other institutions [13]. Also, the survival of this group of patients was significantly reduced if the cytoreduction resulted in tumor greater than 0.25 cm present after surgery. This has been shown in the past by our data and in manuscripts from other institutions [13]. Current data showed that a CT that quantitated concerning CT features had important implications regarding survival of peritoneal mesothelioma patients who had a uniform treatment. This prognostic information regarding survival from the concerning CT features has not been available in the past [4, 5]. Our group published regarding the effects of CT features on completeness of cytoreduction but our current data regarding survival has not been previously published for malignant peritoneal mesothelioma. The clinical value of three assessments of survival (concerning CT features, PCI and CC score) expected following cytoreductive surgery and HIPEC differ greatly in their clinical utility because of the timing of the available information.

Utilization of Concerning CT Features in Other Diseases Treated for Peritoneal Metastases

The 10 concerning CT features used in this study to estimate the survival of malignant peritoneal mesothelioma was a composite of 6 previously reported and 4 specific features for this disease. It is probable that there are well defined CT findings for peritoneal metastases from several different diseases that can estimate the outcome of the malignancy and the available treatments. In our study of the preoperative CT in malignant peritoneal mesothelioma, valuable information became available regarding the survival outcome of this disease. Our success in this project is, we think, related to the uniformity of the disease process, close timing of the CT and the definitive intervention, a uniform treatment plan, and the long-term follow-up available. If a prospective confirmation of these data is sought, all these study criteria would need to be met. A multi-institutional prospective effort to test the utility of preoperative concerning CT features is suggested in a wide variety of diseases with peritoneal metastases.

REFERENCES

[1] Yan TD, Morris DL, Shigeki K, Barrati D, Marcello D. Preoperative investigations in the management of peritoneal surface malignancy with cytoreductive surgery and perioperative intraperitoneal chemotherapy: Expert consensus statement. *J Surg Oncol* 2008;98(4):224-7.

[2] Low RN, Barone RM, Lucero J. Comparison of MRI and CT for predicting the Peritoneal Cancer Index (PCI) preoperatively in patients being considered for cytoreductive surgical procedures. *Ann Surg Oncol* 2015;22(5):1708-15.

[3] van't Sant I, van Eden WJ, Engbersen MP, et al. Diffusion-weighted MRI assessment of the peritoneal cancer index before cytoreductive surgery. *Br J Surg* 2019;4:491-498.

[4] Torkzad MR, Casta N, Bergman A, Ahlström H, Påhlman L, Mahteme H. Comparison between MRI and CT in prediction of peritoneal carcinomatosis index (PCI) in patients undergoing cytoreductive surgery in relation to the experience of the radiologist. *J Surg Oncol* 2015;111:746-51.

[5] Jacquet P, Jelinek JS, Chang D, Koslowe P, Sugarbaker PH. Abdominal computed tomographic scan in the selection of patients with mucinous peritoneal carcinomatosis for cytoreductive surgery. *J Am Coll Surg* 1995;181:530-8.

[6] Yan TD, Haveric N, Carmignani P, Chang D, Sugarbaker PH. Abdominal computed tomography scans in the selection of patients with malignant peritoneal mesothelioma for comprehensive treatment with cytoreductive surgery and perioperative intraperitoneal chemotherapy. *Cancer* 2005;15:839-49.

[7] Rivard JD, Temple WJ, McConnell YJ, et al. Preoperative computed tomography does not predict resectability in peritoneal carcinomatosis. *Am J Surg* 2014;207:760-5.

[8] Sugarbaker PH, Sardi A, Brown G, Dromain C, Rousset P, Jelinek JS. Concerning CT features used to select patients for treatment of peritoneal metastases, a pictoral essay. *Int J Hyperthermia* 2017;33(5):497-504.

[9] Sugarbaker PH, van der Speeten K. An overview of peritonectomy, visceral resection, and therapeutic laparoscopy for peritoneal surface malignancy. (In) Sugarbaker PH (Ed.). *Cytoreductive Surgery & Perioperative Chemotherapy for Peritoneal Surface Malignancy. Textbook and Video Atlas.* 2nd Edition. Cine-Med Publishing: Woodbury, CT, 2017, pp. 17-46.

[10] Van der Speeten K, Stuart OA, Sugarbaker PH. Cancer chemotherapy for peritoneal metastases: Pharmacology and treatment. (In) Sugarbaker PH (Ed). *Cytoreductive Surgery & Perioperative Chemotherapy for Peritoneal Surface Malignancy. Textbook and Video Atlas.* 2nd Edition. Cine-Med Publishing: Woodbury, CT, 2017, pp. 47-82.

[11] Jacquet P, Sugarbaker PH. Current methodologies for clinical assessment of patients with peritoneal carcinomatosis. *J Exp Clin Cancer Res* 1996;15(1):49-58.

[12] Jeune F, Brouquet A, Caramella C, et al. Cardiophrenic angle lymph node is an indicator of metastatic spread but not specifically peritoneal carcinomatosis in colorectal cancer patients: Results of a

prospective validation study in 91 patients. *Eur J Surg Oncol* 2016;42(6):861-8.

[13] Yan TD, Welch L, Black D, Sugarbaker PH. A systematic review on the efficacy of cytoreductive surgery combined with perioperative intraperitoneal chemotherapy for diffuse malignant peritoneal mesothelioma. *Ann Oncol* 2007;18:827-34.

[14] Antman KH, Blum RH, Greenberger JS, et al. Multimodality therapy for malignant mesothelioma based on a study of natural history. *Am J Med* 1980;68:356-62.

[15] Sugarbaker PH, Turaga KK, Alexander HR Jr, Deraco M, Hesdorffer M. Management of malignant peritoneal mesothelioma using cytoreductive surgery and perioperative chemotherapy. *J Oncol Pract* 2016;12(10):928-35.

[16] Elias D, Borget I, Farron M, et al. Prognostic significance of visible cardiophrenic angle lymph nodes in the presence of peritoneal metastases from colorectal cancers. *Eur J Surg Oncol* 2013;39(11):1214-8.

[17] Llanos MD, Sugarbaker PH. Symptoms, signs and radiologic findings in patients having reoperative surgery for malignant peritoneal mesothelioma. *Eur J Surg Oncol* 2017;43:138-43.

[18] Low RN, Barone RM. Combined diffusion-weighted and gadolinium-enhanced MRI can accurately predict the peritoneal cancer index preoperatively in patients being considered for cytoreductive surgical procedures. *Ann Surg Oncol* 2012;19:1394-1401.

[19] da Silva RG, Sugarbaker PH. Analysis of prognostic factors in seventy patients having a complete cytoreduction plus perioperative intraperitoneal chemotherapy for carcinomatosis from colorectal cancer. *J Am Coll Surg* 2006;203(6):878-86.

[20] Sugarbaker PH. Pseudomyxoma peritonei and peritoneal metastases from appendiceal malignancy. (In) Sugarbaker PH (Ed). *Cytoreductive Surgery & Perioperative Chemotherapy for Peritoneal Surface Malignancy. Textbook and Video Atlas.* 2nd Edition. Cine-Med Publishing: Woodbury, CT, 2017, pp. 109-132.

LIST OF CONTRIBUTORS

Gina Brown, MD, FRCR
Royal Marsden and Imperial College, London, UK

Clarisse Dromain, MD, PhD
University Hospital CHUV, Lausanne, Switzerland

James S. Jelinek, MD, FACR
Department of Radiology, MedStar Washington Hospital Center, Washington, DC, USA

Russell N. Low, MD
Department of Radiology, Sharp Memorial Hospital, San Diego, CA, USA

Pascal Rousset, MD, PhD
Le Centre Hospitalier Lyon-Sud, Lyon, France

Paul H. Sugarbaker, MD
Center for Gastrointestinal Malignancies, MedStar Washington Hospital Center, Washington, DC, USA

About the Editors

Paul H. Sugarbaker initiated several projects concerning metastatic disease from colon and rectal cancer in the decade between 1976 and 1986. At the Surgery Branch, National Cancer Institute, he initiated surgical technologies to safely resect liver metastases and determine that a long-term survival occurred in approximately one-third of the patients. Another pattern of metastatic disease was peritoneal metastases. This clinical diagnosis was, at that time, universally fatal. The only treatment was palliative systemic chemotherapy which was rarely beneficial. His early efforts using resection alone seemed to be of little benefit. However, after complete cytoreductive surgery using peritonectomy and visceral resections was invented, and perioperative chemotherapy introduced the outcomes dramatically changed. Also, he focused his efforts on a very small part of the colorectum, the appendix, and saw a huge success with the mucinous appendiceal neoplasms. Patients who were routinely considered terminal and having no viable treatment options were showing a survival greater than 50% at 10 years.

The strategy was applied to malignant peritoneal mesothelioma with similar success. Also, ovarian cancer, gastric cancer, and colorectal cancer peritoneal metastases were targets for safe and effective treatment options.

He has worked over the last four and a half decades to make progress in the prevention and treatment of peritoneal metastases. Approximately 2000 treatment centers are currently operational and achieving great success around the globe. He has brought into this effort all the disciplines within oncology to maximize benefits. The radiologist is now an indispensable part of these efforts. The radiology of peritoneal metastases is challenging but our team of five radiologists have made great progress. Our Nova Science Publishers has printed the current "State of the Art" in the book, *Pictorial Essays in Peritoneal Metastases Imaging: CT, MRI and PET-CT.*

Russell N. Low completed his residency in diagnostic radiology at UCSF in 1990 followed by a body imaging fellowship at Stanford Medical Center. In a career that has spanned over three decades he has become a recognized expert in body MR imaging who has authored 68 peer-reviewed articles and 11 book chapters. Defining new MRI techniques for imaging peritoneal cancer has been his focus for decades. A frequently invited guest speaker Dr. Low has given over 300 educational lectures which convey his passion for body MRI. Always looking and exploring Dr. Low and his staff have helped to define body MRI, optimizing protocols and looking for new and unexpected clinical applications.

INDEX

C

D

E

F

M

Q

R

S

T

U

V